CW00385493

£7·95

NATURE'S

Cosmetic Recipes You Can Make at Home

Collected by Deb Carpenter

Fulcrum Publishing
Golden, Colorado

For my mother, Mary Ann Wellnitz, who is the perfect combination of inner and outer beauty; and to my lovely daughters, Jamie and Jessica.

Copyright © 1995 Deb Carpenter
Cover image © 1995 Mimi Osborne
Book design by Bill Spahr

The author disclaims any liability arising from the use of this book.

All rights reserved. No part of this publication may be reproduced, stored in a retrieval system, or transmitted in any form or by any means, electronic, mechanical, photocopying, recording, or otherwise, without the prior written permission of the publisher.

Library of Congress Cataloging-in-Publication Data
Carpenter, Deb.
    Nature's beauty kit: cosmetic recipes you can make at home/
collected by Deb Carpenter.
        p.   cm.
    Includes bibliographical references and index.
    ISBN 1-55591-221-4 (pbk.: alk. paper)
    1. Cosmetics.   2. Beauty, Personal.   3. Herbal cosmetics.
I. Title.
    RA778.C2168 1995
    646.7'2—dc20   95-32290
                                          CIP

Printed in the United States of America

0 9 8 7 6 5

Fulcrum Publishing
16100 Table Mountain Parkway, Suite 300
Golden, Colorado 80403
303/277-1623 • 800/992-2908
www.fulcrum-books.com

Contents

$\mathcal{A}$CKNOWLEDGMENTS

My introduction to natural cosmetics took place at my cousin's house. The beauty treatment we chose was the "mudpack." It had rained the night before, so we simply went outside and scooped some muck from a puddle into a container. Then we trotted upstairs to work before her bedroom mirror. All went well until Kim slapped on a handful of nature's treasure and discovered a worm on her face.

One would think that would have ended my interest in facials and other natural cosmetics, but my fascination only increased. I began clipping recipes from newspapers and magazines, and I inherited my grandmother's worn clippings as well. When my drawer filled, I decided it was time either to do something with this collection or throw it out. By the time I had tested, adapted, organized, and typed all of these snippets, it became clear that my work should benefit more people than myself.

The compilation of recipes became a self-published spiral-bound book, which was set up to be photocopied. I started with 50 copies, thinking I would be lucky to sell half. Black Hills Staple and Spice of Rapid City, South Dakota, was the first store to carry the book, and owner/manager Bart Dean passed it along to Linda Linchester of Herb 'n' Renewal ™ (Laura, Illinois), who began a one-woman crusade to get this book out there. She not only profiled me in her mail-order catalog, but she also shared names, suggested markets, and put in a personal word with her contacts. When sales reached the 2,000 mark, Linda pitched the book to Fulcrum, and they offered me a contract for the revised edition. Thanks, Linda. Thank you, also, to the Fulcrum staff.

An invaluable source for the revision was Ruth Winter's book, *A Consumer's Dictionary of Cosmetic Ingredients.* Every woman should have a copy of this book on her makeup table.

I am also indebted to our foremothers for trying and testing the variety and mixture of ingredients that found their way into these recipes.

I hope this book will help women of the future care for their bodies in a manner compatible with nature. There is a saying that "taking joy in living is a woman's best cosmetic." That, by far, is the best advice I can offer.

*I*NTRODUCTION

While studying the Lakota culture and their use of plants, I decided to try the yucca root as shampoo. I did exactly as instructed; I dug the root, cut and mashed it, then boiled it in water and used the suds to cleanse my scalp. The minute the liquid touched my skin, I knew I was allergic. It burned fiercely, even after I stuck my head under the showerhead and rinsed out all traces of the yucca. It took a week for the rash to go away. After that experience, I NEVER USE A NEW PRODUCT WITHOUT FIRST TESTING IT.

CAUTION: ALWAYS "PATCH TEST" ANY COSMETIC BEFORE APPLYING TO A LARGER SKIN OR SCALP AREA. YOU MAY BE ALLERGIC TO A PRODUCT, EVEN THOUGH IT IS "NATURAL."

To patch test, apply a small amount of the preparation on the inside of your elbow. Wait 24 hours. If there is no redness or irritation, go ahead and use the product. IF YOU DEVELOP A RASH OR ANY TYPE OF REACTION, DO NOT APPLY THE PRODUCT.

GENERAL INSTRUCTIONS FOR SKIN CARE

I remember once walking out of the grocery store with a small bag. My dad took a peek inside and saw a candy bar and acne medicine.

"Deb," he said, "that's a little like hitting yourself over the head with a hammer and then taking an aspirin."

The point is that what you put inside your body is as important as, if not more important than, what you put on the outside. The best complexions come from a good diet.

Besides your diet, heredity, exercise, lifestyle, stress, nicotine, and general health can affect your complexion. Sun, or lack of sun, also predicts how the skin will look over a lifetime. Sun ages the skin because it dries it and promotes loss of elasticity. Too much sun also puts you at risk for skin cancer. Stay away from burns and deep tans, apply sun block before you go out in the sun and moisturizer when you come in from the sun.

Why does diet matter to our skin? Why should sun and drying make a difference to our skin's elasticity? What is skin, anyway? A miniature science lesson may help explain some of these general rules.

Our skin, hair, nails, and breasts all fall under the physiological category "Integumentary System." What we call "skin" is actually made up of three complex parts. The two top layers are known as the epidermis and dermis, and underneath these is the subcutaneous tissue which makes up the third main part of the skin.

The subcutaneous tissue is a layer of fatty tissue which cushions and protects glands, blood vessels, and the nerves of the upper two layers. This tissue also helps support the skin and gives it its shape. As the layers thin, the skin loosens and sags. As the dermis stretches and thins, sagging increases. Natural aging of these parts of the skin causes wrinkles. Keeping your skin as healthy as possible will help delay the wrinkling process.

The dermis is that connective layer of tissue that separates the epidermis from the subcutaneous tissue. This layer contains blood vessels and nerve endings. It also contains sweat glands which give off water and eliminate wastes. It contains oil glands, too, which lubricate your skin. It is made up mostly of collagen, which is a fibrous protein. The dermis feeds the epidermis. That is why it is as important to monitor your diet as it is to monitor your cosmetic case.

Epi is the Greek prefix which means "on, upon, or in addition to." *Dermis* is derived from the Greek root "derma" or "dermatos," meaning "skin." The epidermis, or top layer of skin, is a thin covering (thicker on the scalp, palms, and soles) that acts as a barrier. It keeps everything in your body that belongs inside and everything out of your body that belongs outside. Bacteria can enter the body through damaged skin, so that's why it is important to take care of it properly. The cells of the epidermis are continually sloughed off, and our outer layer completely renews itself about every seven years. If the dead cells aren't removed daily, the epidermis can become hard and leathery. Also, organisms that grow naturally on the epidermis are more likely to cause infection if the skin is damaged. Those organisms are constantly removed through exfoliation, bathing, and drying. Therefore, developing good skin care habits can prevent illness.

Skin absorbs whatever is put on it. Most shampoos and soaps are alkaline, but the skin is slightly acidic, so it needs acidic products as well. The normal pH of skin ranges from

4.2 to 5.6. pH solutions are measured on a scale of 14 to show whether a product is alkaline or acidic. A neutral product like water measures 7. Anything above 7 is alkaline; below 7 is the acidity your skin needs. Vinegar and lemon juice are acidic. You can test the acidity of products by using litmus paper. Red litmus paper turns blue when it comes in contact with acid.

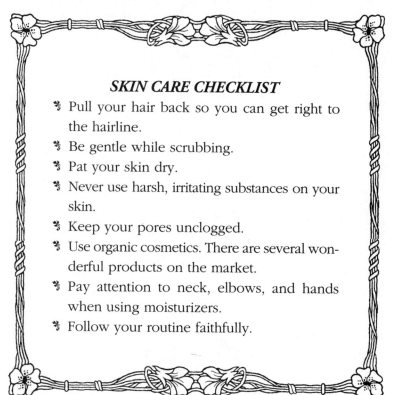

SKIN CARE CHECKLIST

❦ Pull your hair back so you can get right to the hairline.

❦ Be gentle while scrubbing.

❦ Pat your skin dry.

❦ Never use harsh, irritating substances on your skin.

❦ Keep your pores unclogged.

❦ Use organic cosmetics. There are several wonderful products on the market.

❦ Pay attention to neck, elbows, and hands when using moisturizers.

❦ Follow your routine faithfully.

$\mathcal{F}$ACE AND $\mathcal{N}$ECK

You'll need the following items for your morning and nightly rituals:

- Water
- Clean towel
- Clean, soft washcloth
- Cotton balls
- Splasher (page 6–8)
- Oil, soap, or cleansing lotion (page 4–6)
- Moisturizer/night cream (page 8–13)

Morning Ritual

1. Rinse your face with lukewarm water, then splash with cool water at least 12 times. Or, after rinsing your face with lukewarm water, fill a bowl with cold water and a few ice cubes. Hold your breath and dunk your face 4 times, holding your breath as long as possible each time you dunk. This closes your pores and wakes up your skin.
2. Pat your skin dry.
3. Apply splasher.
4. Apply moisturizer, using facial massage technique (pages 2–4).

Nightly Ritual

1. Gently (especially around the eyes) pat oil, cold cream, castile soap, or cleansing lotion to cleanse your skin.
2. Leave cleansing solution on one minute, then gently remove with a soft washcloth that has been soaked in warm water.
3. Rinse thoroughly with cool water. Splash your face at least 12 times.
4. Apply splasher.
5. Apply night cream, using facial massage technique.

Always remember to give your neck the same attention as you do your face. You may want to follow the cleansing of your neck with a nonalcoholic toner stroked on very gently with a cotton ball. This helps slough away dead cells that accumulate on the neck and cause the skin to look dull. Moisturize your neck during your facial massage.

For a special neck cream, add an infusion of sage to your moisturizer.

FACIAL MASSAGE

Before you follow the steps in your morning and nightly rituals, learn a bit more about handling your face. Facial massage can be very beneficial, unless you do it wrong, in which case it can stretch your skin improperly.

Use both hands for daily applications of skin preparations. Use firm pressure at the beginning of the stroke, lightening it as you move upward. If using a liquid preparation, keep fingers well moistened.

It is sometimes helpful to remember the steps by ritualizing the facial massage through prayer. The suggested prayer is in italics. Follow this step-by-step routine in your facial massage:

1. From the outer edge of the collarbone, stroke upward to jaw bone, around the neck; repeat four times.

   I lift my head upward in acknowledgment

2. From beneath the chin, stroke along the jawline up the side of the cheek to the temple; repeat four times on each side of your face.

   Help me to let go of my worries or anger
   and to keep a pleasant countenance

3. From tip of nose, stroke upward to hairline, working on forehead with short strokes to hairline, finishing with brisk cross strokes from center of forehead out, alternating sides of the forehead. Do the cross strokes four times.

   Help me to keep my mind on the important things in life

4. From the outer corner of the mouth, stroke along mouth and nose line to inner corner of the eye; repeat four times.

   Help me to keep my nose out of other people's business
   and to take time to smell the roses

5. To help tighten eyelids, "walk" the pad across the eye-
   brow and on the temples to the upper ear, giving lifting
   pressure with each movement. NEVER work on the eyelid
   itself. Repeat this four times on each side of the face.

   Help me see the world through the eyes of many people,
   not just my own

6. From under the chin, stroke four times toward the mouth,
   then from the center of the chin stroke four times hori-
   zontally toward the jaw edge. From the center of the
   chin, make four circles around the mouth.

   Help me to remember that my words can be helpful or
   harmful, and help me to control those words

CLEANSING LOTIONS

Herbal Cleansing Lotion

Ingredients:
   water, fennel seeds, dried elder flowers, honey,
   buttermilk

Instructions:
1. Boil 1/2 cup of water.
2. Add 1 teaspoon crushed fennel seeds and 1 teaspoon dried
   elder flowers.
3. Let steep for 15 minutes.
4. Strain infusion into a clean jar. *(What is not used in the*
   lotion may be stored in the refrigerator to use as a splasher.)

5. Blend 1 tablespoon cooled infusion with 1 tablespoon honey and 3 tablespoons buttermilk.
6. Pour herbal cleansing lotion into a small container and store in refrigerator.
7. To use, pour a small amount into your hands and warm it before applying to your face. Remove with a wash cloth soaked in warm water, then rinse thoroughly and apply splasher and moisturizer.

Oatmeal Cleansing Lotion

Ingredients:
   oatmeal, water

Instructions:
1. Fill a jar halfway with oatmeal.
2. Fill to the top with water.
3. Let soak for 24 hours, shaking at regular intervals.
4. Pour off water into a clean jar, using it on a cotton ball to cleanse the pores. Discard the oatmeal.

Heavy-Duty Cleanser

USE THIS HEAVY-DUTY CLEANSER ON YOUR FACE ONCE A MONTH.

Ingredients:
   oatmeal, almond meal, water

Instructions:
1. Mix 1 tablespoon oatmeal with 1/2 tablespoon almond meal.

2. Add 1 teaspoon water to moisten.
3. Rub into clean, wet skin, over entire face and neck, with the exception of the eye area.
4. Rinse thoroughly with warm water, then cool.
5. Pat dry.
6. Apply splasher.
7. Apply moisturizer.

SPLASHERS

Mix these ingredients according to directions, then splash them on your face or apply them with a cotton ball as an astringent.

Herbal splashers can be made by steeping fresh or dried herbs in boiling water for 5 to 15 minutes. Another way to prepare the infusion is to put the herbs in cold water in a glass jar and set the jar in the sun. Always refrigerate the herbal splashers and discard unused portion after four days. Remember not to use aluminum containers to make herbal solutions. Dried herbs are more concentrated, so you will only need about a tablespoon per cup. Fresh herbs require about a handful per quart. See the herb chart in the appendix to find the herbs appropriate for your particular need.

Splasher for Normal Skin

Ingredients:
apple cider vinegar, water

Instructions:
1. Mix 1 tablespoon apple cider vinegar with 3 tablespoons water.
2. Splash on face or apply with a cotton ball.

Splasher for Oily Skin

Ingredients:
apple cider vinegar, water

Instructions:
1. Mix 2 tablespoons apple cider vinegar with 2 tablespoons water.
2. Splash on face or apply with a cotton ball.

Cucumber Splasher

Ingredients:
cucumber, water, fresh mint

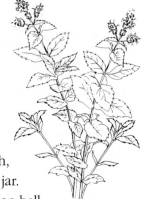

Instructions:
1. Peel and cut half of a cucumber.
2. Mix in blender until smooth.
3. Add an equal amount of water.
4. Add 4 fresh mint leaves.
5. Mix in blender until smooth.
6. Strain through muslin, cheesecloth, or a paper coffee filter into clean jar.
7. Splash on face or apply with a cotton ball.
8. Store in refrigerator, discarding any unused portion after four days.

AUTHOR NOTE: DON'T FORGET TO DO A PATCH TEST. SOME INDIVIDU-
ALS ARE HIGHLY ALLERGIC TO MINT WHEN IT IS APPLIED EXTERNALLY.

Cucumber and Witch Hazel Splasher

Ingredients:
cucumber, witch hazel

Instructions:
1. Peel and cut half of a cucumber.
2. Mix in blender until smooth.
3. Add 2 tablespoons witch hazel.
4. Mix in blender a few seconds.
5. Strain through muslin, cheesecloth, or paper coffee filter into a clean jar.
6. Splash on face or apply with a cotton ball.
7. Store in the refrigerator, discarding any unused portion after four days.

MOISTURIZERS AND NIGHT CREAMS

My youngest daughter, Jessie, was very quiet for a three-year-old. I came into the dining room to see what she was doing and found her sitting on the table, lid off the butter dish, rubbing margarine all over her bare arms and legs. "I'm using moisturizer, Mommy!" What could I say? Here was a child after my own heart.

Dryness is the greatest factor when it comes to skin aging, so use a moisturizer to keep your skin supple and youthful. The oils in the moisturizer recipes tend to clog pores and may cause acne if you have naturally oily skin, so it is important to follow your daily, weekly, and monthly cleansing rituals. It is also important to experiment with lighter oils, different herbal splashers, etc., until you find the right combination for your skin.

The following recipes may feel "greasy" to you at first, but you will soon get used to the products and begin to appreciate the way they leave your skin feeling smooth and soft.

You may want to put the final mixtures in two containers and share one with a friend, or use the products as body moisturizers, over the entire body after you shower or bathe. You may also want to put the butter dish out of reach of your three-year-old....

Aloe Vera Cleanser/Moisturizer

Ingredients:
> aloe vera gel, olive oil (see Appendix A for alternative types), lanolin, beeswax, rose water

Instructions:
1. Mix 1 tablespoon aloe vera gel into 1/3 cup olive oil. Set aside.
2. Melt 2 tablespoons lanolin and 1 tablespoon grated beeswax in a double boiler or microwave. If you are using the microwave, stir at 10-second intervals.
3. Remove from heat or microwave and slowly pour oil/aloe vera mixture into melted lanolin/beeswax mixture, stirring as you pour.
4. Stir in 2 tablespoons rose water.

5. Transfer to blender or mix with an electric hand mixer and blend until mixture is thick and creamy.
6. Pour mixture into a clean, wide-mouth container before it starts to solidify.

Natural Protein Moisturizer

Ingredients:

peanut oil (see Appendix A for alternative types), lanolin, water, lecithin or a whole egg, perfume

Instructions:

1. Blend together 1/2 cup peanut oil with 1 tablespoon lanolin and heat slowly in a double boiler or microwave until lanolin has melted completely. (If using microwave, heat at 30-second intervals until melted.)
2. Add 1/3 cup water and a whole egg (beaten) or 1 tablespoon lecithin in place of the egg. Beat with hand mixer until smooth.
3. Simmer a few minutes or put back in the microwave until the mixture has thickened. (If using the microwave, heat at 15 second intervals, stirring at each interval.)
4. Beat with hand mixer and add a few drops of your favorite perfume to overpower the odor of the lanolin. Put mixture in a container and refrigerate.

AUTHOR NOTE: THIS MIXTURE NEEDS TO SIMMER IN ORDER FOR IT TO THICKEN. I TRIED IT WITH LIQUID LANOLIN, SKIPPING STEP 3, AND DID NOT HAVE GOOD RESULTS. THE MOISTURIZER SHOULD KEEP FOR UP TO THREE WEEKS IN THE REFRIGERATOR.

Night Cream/Moisturizer

Ingredients:

egg, oils (almond, sunflower, corn, or coconut), lemon juice, cider vinegar, additives (optional)

Instructions:

1. Using an electric mixer or blender, blend together 1 egg (room temperature) and 1/4 cup almond oil (sesame oil may be substituted), beating at low speed until thoroughly combined.
2. Slowly add 1/4 cup sunflower oil (may substitute safflower oil) while running the blender or mixer.
3. Slowly add 1 tablespoon lemon juice and 1/2 tablespoon cider vinegar while running the blender or mixer. If you are using herbal additives, the herbal vinegars may be substituted for plain cider vinegar.
4. When the mixture is thoroughly blended, slowly add 1/4 cup corn oil (avocado oil may be substituted) and then 1/4 cup coconut oil. These oils should both be added while running the blender or mixer.
5. Blend until thick. If mixture doesn't thicken, refrigerate and then blend again.
6. Add drops of perfume if desired. If you are using other additives, blend them in at this point. (See the following section.)
7. Refrigerate. Discard after 2 weeks.

AUTHOR NOTE: YOU MAY WANT TO EXPERIMENT WITH THE OILS, DEPENDING ON YOUR SKIN TYPE. USE LIGHTER OILS FOR OILY SKIN. THIS RECIPE MAKES ABOUT 8 OUNCES OF NIGHT CREAM/MOISTURIZER AND CAN BE HALVED BEFORE BLENDING IN THE ADDITIVES TO MAKE SPECIFIC TYPES OF CREAM.

Additives

Aloe vera—Add 1 tablespoon aloe vera gel per 4 ounces of night cream.

Herbs—See Appendix B for information regarding herbal additives. The rule of thumb is to make an infusion of 1 to 3 tablespoons per cup of hot water. Let the herbs steep in the hot water for about 10 minutes. After straining off the herbs and letting cool, add 1 tablespoon of this infusion to 4 ounces of night cream after it is completely blended. This will make the cream more of a lotion. If you like the thick consistency, infuse the herbs in the vinegar.

To infuse the herbs in vinegar, place a dried sprig or 1 table-spoon of the herb in a sterile glass spice jar. Heat 1/3 cup vinegar in the microwave until it is hot but not boiling and pour heated vinegar over the herbs. Put the cap on loosely, until cooled. (Lid should be glass or plastic, because the acid in vinegar reacts with metal.) When cool, seal tightly and put in a dark place for 1 to 3 weeks, shaking every day. Before using, strain off liquid through muslin or cheesecloth and discard the herbs.

Lecithin—Lecithin helps rebuild cells. Add 1 tablespoon liquid lecithin per 4 ounces of night cream. Since lecithin is found naturally in raw egg yolks, you may add 3 beaten egg yolks per 4 ounces of night cream. Discard unused portion after one week if using egg yolks.

Vitamin A—This vitamin is said to help to lubricate and heal the skin. It is best to only add a few (1 to 5) drops per 4 ounces of night cream, since too much vitamin A can cause the skin to turn a yellowish color. Do not use vitamin A as an additive if you are pregnant, because too high of levels may cause birth defects. Add vitamin A to your diet by eating green and yellow vegetables such as carrots, spinach, pumpkin, and also foods such as cantaloupe, liver, and cod liver oil.

Vitamin C—Vitamin C is good for the skin and helps heal cuts. As a dietary aid, try eating citrus fruits, broccoli, and green peppers.

Vitamin D—Since vitamin D helps your body absorb calcium, it is essential for strong bones and teeth. Vitamin D is also good for the hair and prevents aging of the skin. The best way to use vitamin D cosmetically is to make sure you have it in your diet. Sources of vitamin D are fish, milk, cheese, and yogurt. You also need a certain amount of sunlight for your body to manufacture vitamin D.

Vitamin E—Vitamin E promotes elasticity of the skin and is a natural healing agent as well. Many people use vitamin E oil on burns. While I was pregnant, I used vitamin E oil on my breasts and tummy daily, and my stretch marks are virtually nonexistent. Add up to 1 teaspoon per 4 ounces of night cream. Also add vitamin E to your diet by including eggs, wheat germ, whole grains, broccoli, leafy greens, and vegetable oils.

GET STEAMED

Steam your skin once a week to clean the pores, increase surface blood flow, and moisturize the skin. Add herbs to make it more soothing and/or stimulating. (See Appendix B for suggestions. These herbs can be used alone or in combination. Remember to patch test the herbs before using them in a facial steam.)

1. Pull your hair back, then clean your face thoroughly.
2. Fill a bowl half full of boiling water. Carefully cover your face and the bowl with a large towel, taking care to prevent burns.
3. Steam your face for 10 minutes.
4. Remove the towel and splash your face 12 times with lukewarm water.
5. Pat dry.
6. Apply a facial mask (pages 16–35).
7. After facial mask is removed, apply splasher and moisturizer.

CAUTION: FACIAL STEAMS ARE NOT RECOMMENDED FOR PEOPLE WITH VERY DRY SKIN, ASTHMA, BREATHING DIFFICULTIES, OR DILATED FACIAL VEINS. SEE PAGE 35 FOR A SAFE FACIAL MASK FOR PEOPLE WITH DILATED FACIAL VEINS.

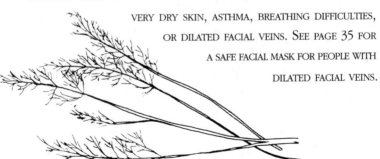

Herbal Facial Steam 1

Ingredients:

fennel seeds, dried mint, dried sage, dried elder flowers, powdered licorice root, water. See Appendix B for additional or substitute herbs.

Instructions:

1. Crush 1 tablespoon fennel seeds and place in a large bowl.
2. Add 1 tablespoon dried mint, 2 tablespoons dried sage, 1 tablespoon dried elder flowers, 1 tablespoon powdered licorice root. Mix herbs together with hands.
3. Pour 1 quart boiling water over the herbs.
4. Put your face over the bowl, covering your head with a towel to form a tent. Keep your face above the bowl about 12 inches.
5. Steam your face for 5 to 10 minutes and relax. Relaxing is the hardest part. You may want to listen to a book on tape or your favorite CD. To give the steam a boost, blow across the surface of the water every now and then.
6. Splash your face with cool water 12 times and pat dry.
7. Apply a facial mask or apply moisturizer to lock in the moisture.

AUTHOR NOTE: YOU MAY WANT TO STRAIN OFF THE HERBS AND SAVE THE INFUSION, WHICH CAN BE ADDED TO YOUR FACIAL MASKS (1 TABLESPOON FOR MOST RECIPES). THE REMAINDER OF THE INFUSION CAN BE KEPT AT ROOM TEMPERATURE AND USED TO RINSE THE DRIED FACIAL MASK FROM YOUR FACE BEFORE SPLASHING WITH COOL WATER.

Herbal Facial Steam 2

Ingredients:
> dried bay leaves, dried chamomile flowers, dried rosemary, fresh rose petals, water

Instructions:
1. Place 4 dried bay leaves, 1 tablespoon dried chamomile flowers, 1 tablespoon dried rosemary, and 1 handful fresh rose petals in a bowl.
2. Pour 1 quart boiling water over herbs.
3. Put your face over the bowl, covering your head with a towel to form a tent. Keep your face above the bowl about 12 inches.
4. Steam your face 5 to 10 minutes. It can be difficult to steam for this long, but try and relax. My favorite way to combat this problem is to listen to a good country music station and blow across the water in time to the music, trying to make patterns with the floating herbs. (All right, then, come up with your own idea....)
5. Splash your face with cool water 12 times and pat dry.
6. Apply a facial mask OR apply moisturizer to lock in the moisture.

PUT ON A MASK

Once when my husband was working late and my toddlers were in bed, I decided to experiment with a facial mask. After applying one, I decided to relax on the waterbed in a darkened room rather than in the tub.

My four-year-old got up and wandered into the room. After a startled look at me, she asked, "Mommy, what do you have on your face?"

"Oatmeal and honey, Sweetheart."

"Why did you put it on your face instead of in your mouth, Mommy?"

"It's a face mask. It's supposed to make Mommy pretty."

"Mommy, I don't think you look very pretty."

This section is dedicated to you, Jamie.

Your face must be clean before you begin, so cleanse it thoroughly and then "get steamed." Since most of the facial masks remain 10 to 30 minutes, you may want to treat yourself to a bath while your facial is at work. Remember to treat the oily parts of your skin separately from the dry parts. Most people have an oily T zone that consists of the forehead, nose, and chin.

When you combine herbs with oil, oatmeal, clay, or yogurt and apply these masks to your face, you are nourishing your skin in the simplest manner. See Appendix B for suggestions on herbs appropriate to use in facial masks. Use a facial mask every week.

The following recipes are grouped according to skin type, from dry to normal to oily, with special problems at the end of the section.

Banana Facial Mask for Dry Skin

Ingredients:

banana, sunflower oil

Instructions:

1. Mash half of a banana.
2. Add 2 tablespoons sunflower oil.
3. Mash or blend well.
4. Apply the mixture to your clean face.
5. Leave on 20 minutes.
6. Rinse with warm water, then cool water.
7. Pat dry.

Herbal Oil Mask for Dry Skin

Ingredients:

avocado oil, borage flowers

Instructions:

1. During the morning, fill a small, sterile spice jar with avocado oil.
2. Add 12 fresh borage flowers to the oil.
3. Let the jar stand in the summer sun for the day, then remove the borage flowers.
4. Using cotton balls, apply the oil to your clean face.
5. Leave on 10 to 15 minutes.
6. Rinse with warm water, then cool water.

Oatmeal Facial Mask for Dry Skin

Ingredients:

egg yolk, honey, milk or yogurt, uncooked oatmeal, almond meal

Instructions:

1. Mix 1 egg yolk and 1 tablespoon honey. Set aside.
2. Mix together 1 tablespoon oatmeal and 1 tablespoon almond meal.
3. Stir the egg mixture into the meal mixture.
4. Add 1 tablespoon milk or yogurt.
5. Apply the mixture to your face and allow it to dry completely (approximately 20 to 30 minutes).
6. Wash with a cloth soaked in warm water.
7. Rinse with warm water, then cool water.
8. Pat dry, then apply splasher and moisturizer.

Oatmeal Facial Mask to Soften Rough, Dry Skin

Ingredients:

flaxseed, water, uncooked oatmeal, almond meal

Instructions:

1. Heat 1 teaspoon flaxseed in 1/2 cup water and stir constantly until it thickens.
2. Strain liquid off and add 1/4 cup to a mix of 1 tablespoon uncooked oatmeal and 1 tablespoon almond meal.
3. Spread the paste on cleansed face and let dry for 20 minutes.
4. Wash face with a soft cloth that has been soaked in lukewarm water.

5. Splash face with lukewarm water, then cool water.
6. Pat dry.
7. Apply splasher, then moisturizer.

Apricot Facial Mask for Normal Skin

Ingredients:
apricots (fresh or dry)

Instructions:
1. Mash 2 to 4 apricots (if using dry apricots, soak 4 of them for 2 hours in just enough water to cover them, and then mash them).
2. Spread on the face and wait 20 minutes.
3. Rinse thoroughly with warm water, then cool water.
4. Pat dry.
5. Apply splasher, then moisturizer or night cream.

Beer Facial Mask for Normal Skin

HOPS ARE SUPPOSED TO HAVE A HEALING EFFECT ON THE SKIN AND BE VERY STIMULATING TO IT. SOME PEOPLE, HOWEVER, ARE ALLERGIC TO HOPS, SO BE SURE TO DO A PATCH TEST FIRST.

Ingredients:
beer

Instructions:
1. Apply beer externally.
2. Leave on for 15 minutes.
3. Rinse and pat dry.
4. Apply moisturizer or night cream.

Fennel Facial Mask for Normal Skin

Ingredients:

fennel seeds, water, honey, yogurt

Instructions:

1. Make a fennel seed infusion by pouring 1/2 cup boiling water over 1 tablespoon crushed fennel seeds. Let this steep for 10 minutes. Strain. Let cool.
2. Mix 1 tablespoon honey with 1 tablespoon yogurt.
3. Add 1 teaspoon cooled fennel seed infusion to the honey and yogurt mixture. Stir.
4. Spread the mixture on face and neck.
5. After 15 minutes, rinse off with warm, then cool water. You may use leftover fennel seed infusion as a splasher.
6. Follow with a moisturizer.

    AUTHOR NOTE: YOU MAY SUBSTITUTE THE LEFTOVER INFUSION FROM THE HERBAL CLEANSING LOTION, IN WHICH CASE YOU WILL START WITH STEP 2.

Oatmeal Facial Mask for Normal Skin

Ingredients:

water, dried rosemary leaves, uncooked oatmeal, almond meal

Instructions:

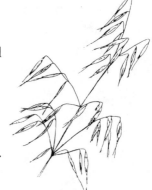

1. Pour 1/2 cup boiling water over 1 teaspoon dried rosemary leaves.
2. Steep for 15 minutes, then strain.

3. In a separate bowl, mix together 1 tablespoon uncooked oatmeal and 1 tablespoon almond meal.

4. Add enough rosemary infusion to make a thick paste. (Refrigerate leftover infusion to use as a splasher.)

5. Spread the paste on cleansed face, but DO NOT PUT PASTE ON YOUR EYES OR LIPS.

6. After 20 minutes, wash face with a soft cloth which has been soaked in lukewarm water.

7. Splash face with lukewarm water, then cool water.

8. Pat dry.

9. Apply rosemary splasher, then moisturizer.

Buttermilk Facial Mask for Oily Skin

Ingredients:

buttermilk (room temperature)

Instructions:

1. Apply buttermilk.

2. Leave on for 15 minutes.

3. Rinse thoroughly with warm water, then cool water.

4. Pat dry.

5. Apply splasher.

6. Apply moisturizer.

Egg White Facial Mask for Oily Skin

Ingredients:

egg white

Instructions:

1. Beat 1 egg white.
2. Apply to your face, especially the T zone.
3. Leave on for 15 minutes.
4. Rinse thoroughly with warm water, then cool water.
5. Pat dry.
6. Apply splasher.
7. Apply moisturizer.

Herbal Facial Mask for Oily Skin

Ingredients:

dried yarrow, water, honey, yogurt

Instructions:

1. Make a yarrow infusion by pouring boiling water over 1 tablespoon dried yarrow leaves and flowers. Let this steep for 10 minutes. Strain. Let cool.
2. Mix 1 tablespoon honey with 1 tablespoon yogurt.
3. Add 1 teaspoon cooled yarrow infusion to the honey and yogurt mixture. Stir.
4. Spread the mixture on face and neck.
5. After 15 minutes, rinse off with warm water, then cool water. (You may use leftover yarrow infusion as a splasher.)
6. Follow with a moisturizer.

Herbs and Earth Facial Pack for Oily Skin

Ingredients:

water, dried lemongrass, dried sage, yogurt, Fuller's Earth

Instructions:

1. Simmer 1 teaspoon dried lemongrass and 1 teaspoon dried sage in 2 cups water for 15 minutes. (Use a glass pot or a glass jar in a pan of water.)
2. While waiting for the solution to heat, mix 1 teaspoon yogurt with 1 teaspoon honey (both feed and clear the skin).
3. Add 1 teaspoon Fuller's Earth to the yogurt and honey mixture. Stir.
4. While herbs are simmering, you may want to indulge in a steam facial by standing over the stove. Be careful to stay far enough away so that you don't get burned.
5. After herbs have simmered for 15 minutes, strain off the liquid through muslin or cheesecloth. Let cool.
6. Add 1 teaspoon of herbal infusion to the yogurt, honey, and Fuller's Earth mixture. Stir.
7. Apply the pack to your face and neck with your fingers. Do not apply to the eye area.
8. Let this mixture dry for 20 minutes.
9. Remove by splashing your face and neck with warm water, gradually cooling to tepid. Pat dry, apply splasher and moisturizer.

   Author note: This mask shouldn't be used more than once a month. The skin's oil glands are stimulated when too much oil is depleted, so using it too often defeats the purpose.

Meal Facial Mask for Oily Skin

Ingredients:
cornmeal, almond meal, water

Instructions:
1. Mix 1 tablespoon cornmeal with 1 tablespoon almond meal.
2. Add water to make a paste.
3. Apply.
4. After 15 minutes, rinse thoroughly with warm water, then cool water.
5. Pat dry.
6. Apply splasher.
7. Apply moisturizer.

Oatmeal Facial Mask for Oily Skin

Ingredients:
water, dried yarrow, uncooked oatmeal, almond meal

Instructions:
1. Pour 1/2 cup boiling water over 1 teaspoon dried yarrow.
2. Steep for 15 minutes, then strain.
3. In a separate bowl, mix together 1 tablespoon uncooked oatmeal and 1 tablespoon almond meal.
4. Add enough yarrow infusion to make a thick paste. (Refrigerate leftover infusion to use as a splasher.)
5. SPREAD THE PASTE ON CLEANSED FACE, BUT DO NOT PUT ON EYES OR LIPS.
6. After 20 minutes, wash face with a soft cloth that has been soaked in lukewarm water.

7. Splash face with lukewarm water, then cool water.
8. Pat dry.
9. Apply yarrow splasher, then moisturizer.

Stimulating Oatmeal Pack for Oily Skin

Ingredients:

boiling water, dried peppermint, dried elder flowers, un-cooked oatmeal, almond meal

Instructions:

1. Pour 1 cup boiling water over 1 teaspoon dried peppermint and 1 teaspoon dried elder flowers. Let steep for 10 minutes, then strain.
2. Mix 1 1/2 tablespoons uncooked oatmeal to 1 tablespoon almond meal.
3. Add enough of the peppermint and elder flower infusion to make a workable paste.
4. Spread the warm (not hot) mixture over your face.
5. Let the mixture dry for 20 to 30 minutes.
6. Wash your face with a soft cloth that has been soaked in lukewarm water (you may use the leftover herbal infusion to soak the wash cloth the first time). Continue rinsing your washcloth and using fresh lukewarm water to wash your face until all of the oatmeal has been removed.
7. Splash your face with lukewarm water, then cool water.
8. Pat dry.
9. Apply splasher and moisturizer.

Wheat Germ Mask for Oily Skin

Ingredients:

wheat germ, yogurt

Instructions:

1. Mix 1 tablespoon wheat germ with 1 tablespoon yogurt.
2. Let the mixture stand for a few minutes until it is room temperature.
3. Apply generously to face and neck.
4. Leave on for 15 minutes.
5. Remove with a wash cloth soaked in warm water.
6. Splash your face with lukewarm water, then cool water.
7. Pat dry.
8. Apply splasher and moisturizer.

MASKS FOR SPECIAL PROBLEMS

Bran Facial Mask for Blemishes

Ingredients:

bran, water

Instructions:

1. Mix 2 tablespoons bran with enough warm water to make a paste the desired consistency.
2. Apply to face and leave on for 20 minutes.
3. Rinse thoroughly with warm water, then cool water.
4. Pat dry.
5. Apply splasher.
6. Apply moisturizer.

Buttermilk and Mint Facial Mask for Blemishes

Ingredients:

castor oil, water, dried spearmint, buttermilk, egg white

Instructions:

1. Spread a thin film of castor oil on your clean face. Let dry while performing step 2.
2. Make a spearmint infusion by pouring 1/2 cup boiling water over 1 teaspoon of dried spearmint. Let steep for 5 minutes, then strain.
3. Whisk together 2 tablespoons buttermilk, one egg white, and 1 teaspoon spearmint infusion.
4. Apply to face and leave on for 20 minutes.
5. Rinse thoroughly. Pat dry.
6. Apply splasher and moisturizer.

Honey and Herb Facial Mask to Draw Out Blackheads

Ingredients:

dried sage, water, honey (known for its drawing power), oatmeal, egg white

Instructions:

1. Pour 1/2 cup boiling water over 1 teaspoon dried sage. Let steep for 15 minutes, then strain. Refrigerate.
2. Make a paste of 3 tablespoons oatmeal and 2 tablespoons warm honey.
3. Add 1 teaspoon sage infusion. Save the rest for a splasher.
4. Beat 1 egg white. Fold it in to the meal, honey, and sage mixture.

5. Apply and leave on for 15 minutes.
6. Rinse thoroughly with warm water, then cool water.
7. Pat dry.
8. Apply sage splasher.
9. Apply moisturizer.

AUTHOR NOTE: THIS IS A RUNNY MIX, SO YOU MAY WANT TO APPLY IT DURING YOUR BATH.

Honey and Wheat Germ Facial Mask for Blemishes

Ingredients:

honey (known for its drawing power), wheat germ, vitamin E oil

Instructions:

1. Blend together 1 tablespoon honey with 1 tablespoon wheat germ and a few drops of vitamin E oil.
2. Apply to face, except around eye area, and leave on for 10 minutes.
3. To rinse, splash your face several times with warm water and then scrub your face with mask residue, splashing again to remove.
4. Pat dry.
5. Apply splasher and moisturizer.

AUTHOR NOTE: THIS MAKES A VERY THICK PASTE THAT CAN BE APPLIED TO THE FACE WITH A SPATULA OR PLASTIC KNIFE. EVEN THOUGH IT IS THICK, IT TENDS TO GRAVITATE, SO IS BEST USED DURING A RELAXING BATH.

Honey Facial Mask for Blemishes

Ingredients:

honey (known for its drawing power)

Instructions:

1. Apply warm (not hot) honey to your face.
2. Leave on for 15 minutes.
3. Rinse thoroughly with warm water, then cool water.
4. Pat dry.
5. Apply splasher.
6. Apply moisturizer.

Milk and Honey Facial Mask for Blemishes

Ingredients:

milk, honey (known for its drawing power), egg

Instructions:

1. Mix together 1 tablespoon whole milk, 1 egg, and 1 table-spoon honey. Warm to room temperature.
2. Apply to your face and leave on for 20 minutes or until hardened.
3. Rinse thoroughly with warm water, then cool water.
4. Pat dry.
5. Apply splasher.
6. Apply moisturizer.

AUTHOR NOTE: THIS RECIPE MAKES MORE THAN ONE FACE CAN USE, SO I TREAT MY DOG TO THE REMAINDER, AND WE'RE BOTH HAPPY.

Meal Mask to Draw Out Blackheads

Ingredients:
    oatmeal, almond meal, egg white, water

Instructions:
1. Mix 1/4 cup oatmeal with 2 tablespoons almond meal.
2. Add 1 egg white. Mix well.
3. If mix is too thick, add a few drops of water until you get the consistency you want.
4. Apply thickly to face, omitting the area around the eyes.
5. Leave on for 15 minutes.
6. Rinse thoroughly, then pat dry.
7. Apply splasher and moisturizer.

Tomato Facial Mask to Draw out Blackheads

Ingredients:
    tomato

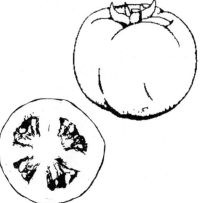

Instructions:
1. Rub affected areas with a slice of raw tomato (this helps restore acidity to your skin's surface).
2. Rinse and pat dry.
3. Apply moisturizer.

Citrus Facial Mask for Blotchy or Discolored Skin

Ingredients:

egg white, frozen concentrated orange juice, lemon juice

Instructions:

1. Beat 1 egg white.
2. Whisk in 1/4 teaspoon frozen concentrated orange juice and 1/2 teaspoon lemon juice.
3. Apply with cotton ball and leave on for 20 minutes.
4. Rinse by splashing face with warm water, then cool water.
5. Pat dry.
6. Apply moisturizer.

Facial Mask for Blotchy or Discolored Skin 1

Ingredients:

yogurt

Instructions:

1. Apply yogurt to face.
2. Leave on overnight.
3. Perform normal morning ritual.

Facial Mask for Blotchy or Discolored Skin 2

Ingredients:

buttermilk

Instructions:

1. Apply room temperature buttermilk to face.
2. Leave on for 20 minutes.

3. Rinse with cool water.
4. Apply moisturizer.

   AUTHOR NOTE: BUTTERMILK IS A NATURAL ASTRINGENT, SO YOU DON'T NEED TO APPLY SPLASHER.

Facial Mask for Flaky Skin

Ingredients:

papaya

Instructions:

1. Mash a wedge of papaya.
2. Apply to the face.
3. Leave on for 15 minutes.
4. Remove from the face with a washcloth that has been soaked in warm water.
5. Rinse by splashing with warm water, then cool water.
6. Pat dry.
7. Apply splasher.
8. Apply moisturizer.

Facial Mask to Fade Freckles

Ingredients:

buttermilk (milk or yogurt can be substituted), dried horse-radish root

Instructions:

1. Apply moisturizer to face.
2. Mix 1 tablespoon buttermilk with 1/2 teaspoon grated dried horseradish root.

3. Let sit for 5 minutes, so dried horseradish has a chance to rehydrate.
4. Apply to face, over top of the moisturizer.
5. Leave on for 10 minutes.
6. Rinse with cool water.
7. Reapply moisturizer.

AUTHOR NOTE: THE HORSERADISH MAKES YOUR SKIN TINGLE, SO IT IS IMPORTANT TO PROTECT YOUR SKIN WITH A LAYER OF MOISTURIZER. IF YOU EXPERIENCE A BURNING SENSATION, RINSE OFF THE HORSERADISH IMMEDIATELY.

Facial Mask to Reduce Large Pores 1

Ingredients:
oatmeal, egg

Instructions:
1. Mix 1 whole egg with 4 tablespoons uncooked oatmeal.
2. Let sit for 5 minutes, then apply generously to face.
3. Leave on for 15 minutes.
4. Remove with washcloth soaked in warm water.
5. Rinse thoroughly with warm water, then cool water.
6. Pat dry.
7. Apply splasher.
8. Apply moisturizer.

Facial Mask to Reduce Large Pores 2

Ingredients:

almond meal, water

Instructions:

1. Mix 2 tablespoons almond meal with enough warm water to make a paste of the desired consistency.
2. Apply generously to face.
3. Leave on 20 minutes.
4. Remove with a washcloth that has been soaked in warm water.
5. Rinse thoroughly with warm water, then cool water.
6. Pat dry.
7. Apply splasher.
8. Apply moisturizer.

Facial Mask for Dilated Veins

Ingredients:

milk

Instructions:

1. Bathe your face in a bowl of tepid milk.
2. Leave on until it dries.
3. Rinse in lukewarm water and pat dry.

   AUTHOR NOTE: IF YOU HAVE DILATED VEINS IN YOUR FACE, YOU SHOULD NEVER USE A FACE PACK OR EXTREMES OF HOT OR COLD.

OTHER SOLUTIONS TO SPECIAL PROBLEMS

The following pages deal with solutions to miscellaneous problems. Acne, blemishes, freckles, etc., have been dealt with in the section on facials, but the following remedies are not facial steams or masks.

Acne

At each meal, take one capsule of each with a large glass of water: alfalfa leaves, kelp, dandelion root. If you prefer teas, combine equal amounts of the herbs in a tea bag or ball, pour boiling water over the herbs, let steep for a few minutes, and drink at each meal.

These herbs are a nutritional aid for acne and should be assisted in their performance by following a healthy diet. It is also important to perform ritual cleansing, steaming, and facial masks.

Blemishes

Rub the blemish or entire face with equal parts cornmeal and oatmeal (dry or as a paste to make a scrub). Rinse thoroughly, first with warm water, then cool water. Pat dry and apply splasher and moisturizer.

Blotchy or Discolored Skin

After cleansing the skin, rub the inside peel of a lemon rind into the area of skin that is blotchy or discolored. Apply moisturizer, since lemon is a drying agent.

Bruises

Mix 1 cup papaya juice with 1 cup pineapple juice. Drink all but 1 or 2 teaspoons, which you can gently rub into the bruised area.

Do this several times a day.

Dry Skin

Mix 1 tablespoon milk and 1 tablespoon butter. Apply to skin and leave on overnight.

Freckles

Pour 1/2 cup boiling water over 1 teaspoon anise seed. Let steep for 15 minutes, then strain. Cool. After it is cooled, dab the infusion onto your face with a cotton ball, splash it on liberally, or put in a spritz bottle and apply several times a day. Keep refrigerated; discard unused portion after four days.

Liver Spots

Use odorless castor oil, vitamin E oil, wheat germ oil, alone or in combination, rubbing the oil onto the spots as often as you think of doing so.

Moles

It is best not to treat moles, but do keep an eye on them. If they change in color or texture, see your physician or dermatologist.

Splotchiness

The Lakota people used juice from wild strawberries to keep the skin smooth and fair. It was believed to reduce splotchiness.

Today, strawberry juice is used in many natural cosmetics as it is reputed to nourish and soften the skin.

Sunburn Treatments

❧ Cool baths or showers help take the heat out.

❧ Mix 1/4 cup vinegar and 1/4 cup water together, then gently spread over the affected areas.

❧ Make a strong solution of black tea. Cool the tea and apply to your skin.

❧ Put one chamomile tea bag in the bottom of a glass jar. Cover with 2 tablespoons witch hazel. Let soak for 15 minutes, then take out the tea bag. Add 1 egg white and 1 teaspoon honey. Use the tea bag like a cotton ball to dab the solution onto the burned areas. Refrigerate and use frequently. Discard any unused portion af ter four days.

Warts

Native Americans used the sap of the milkweed to treat warts, rubbing the liquid onto affected areas until they cleared up.

Warts seem to be caused by a virus that comes and goes at will. They often disappear on their own. Often, any treatment that you seriously believe will work will do the magic for you. Therefore, rub the affected areas with milkweed sap or vitamin E oil four times a day for 12 successive days. (If this doesn't work, dip the wart in stumpwater after dark during a new moon, then throw a dead cat over your left shoulder!)

Wrinkles

Dryness, thinning of the skin, and loss of elasticity are among the reasons skin gets wrinkled. Oils and moisture have to be restored to rejuvenate the skin. The following recipes are for the purpose of restoring moisture and plumping the skin to soften wrinkle lines.

For additional help, use additives in your night cream.

- ❧ Melt 1 tablespoon of lanolin in 1/2 cup almond oil. Blend well. Apply to skin. Leave on for 30 minutes, then gently blot off. Apply often.
- ❧ Spread cocoa butter on generously. Use as often as you like.
- ❧ Beat 1 egg white slightly. Add enough whipping cream so you can apply it easily. Leave on for 30 minutes, then rinse off with lukewarm water and pat dry.

$\mathcal{E}\overline{\textit{YES}}$

The skin surrounding your eyes is the thinnest and most delicate of the body. This causes it to be susceptible to wrinkles and bags. Factors that promote the wrinkling process are squinting, rubbing your eyes, makeup and smoke irritation, and exposure to ultraviolet rays.

Never go to bed with makeup on. Apply a gentle remover to a cotton ball. Press the cotton to the eye, gently, for 5 seconds, then slowly stroke downward. Rinse eyes with lukewarm water, then apply moisturizer or night cream.

When you apply moisturizer to your eye area, NEVER rub it in, but apply it by patting a few dots of cream from the inner corner of the eye to the temple along the eye socket bone and onto the brow bone.

The most effective beauty secret for the eyes is to get lots of rest and to eat foods rich in vitamin A. If you do much close work, such as reading, sewing, or working with computers, remember to give your eyes a break every 5 to 15 minutes. Look up from your work often, glance out a window, close your eyes for a few seconds, or whatever works best for you.

The following remedies are for overstressed eyes, but remember that before you treat your eyes, always clean your eye area gently with your cleanser, then rinse with lukewarm water and blot dry.

AUTHOR NOTE: ALWAYS PATCH TEST THE WASHES OR COMPRESSES BEFORE USING THEM ON THE EYE AREA. THE EYEWASHES ARE HERBAL SOLUTIONS THAT

CAN ALSO BE USED AS COMPRESSES. WHEN USING THEM AS COMPRESSES TO RELIEVE SWOLLEN EYES, SIMPLY DIP A COTTON BALL INTO THE SOLUTION AND APPLY TO YOUR EYELIDS.

EYEWASHES AND COMPRESSES

Chamomile Eyewash

Ingredients:

chamomile, water

Instructions:

1. Simmer 1 teaspoon chamomile in 2 cups water for 5 minutes.
2. Strain and cool the decoction.
3. Bathe the eyes or place soaked cotton balls on eyelids for 5 minutes.
4. Store unused portion in a sterile jar and keep refrigerated. Throw out unused portion after four days.

Eyebright Compress

Ingredients:

eyebright flowers, water

Instructions:

1. Add 1 teaspoon eyebright flowers to 1 cup water.
2. Bring to a boil and simmer for 3 minutes.
3. Strain and cool the decoction.
4. Place soaked cotton balls on eyelids for 5 minutes.
5. Store unused portion in a sterile jar and keep refrigerated. Throw out unused portion after four days.

Fennel Eyewash

Ingredients:
fennel seeds, water

Instructions:
1. Crush 1/2 teaspoon fennel seeds.
2. Simmer fennel seeds in 1 cup water for 3 minutes.
3. Strain and cool the decoction.
4. Bathe the eyes or place soaked cotton balls on eyelids for 5 minutes.
5. Store unused portion in a sterile jar and keep refrigerated. Throw out unused portion after four days.

Herbal Combination Eyewash

Ingredients:
fennel seeds, eyebright, chamomile, water

Instructions:
1. Crush 1/2 teaspoon fennel seeds, mix with 1/2 teaspoon eyebright and 1/2 teaspoon chamomile.
2. Simmer this combination of herbs in 2 cups water for 5 minutes.
3. Strain and cool the decoction.
4. Bathe the eyes or place soaked cotton balls on eyelids for 5 minutes.
5. Store unused portion in a sterile jar and keep refrigerated. Throw out unused portion after four days.

Ice Milk Compress

Ingredients:

milk, water, ice cubes

Instructions:

1. Combine 1/4 cup milk with 1/4 cup water.
2. Add ice cubes.
3. Saturate a soft cloth with the mixture and apply it to your eyes for 5 to 10 minutes while lying down.

Parsley Compress

Ingredients:

parsley, water

Instructions:

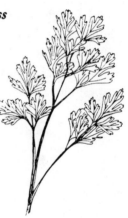

1. Pour boiling water over 2 tea-spoons fresh parsley and allow it to steep for 15 minutes.
2. Cool and strain.
3. Soak cotton balls in the infusion and place on eyes for 15 minutes to relieve puffiness.

Potato Compress

Ingredients:

raw potato

Instructions:

1. Peel and grate half a raw potato onto a soft, wet cloth.

2. Apply this to your eyelids for 10 minutes.
3. Be sure to peel away all potato fragments and rinse your eyes gently with lukewarm water, or the potato may leave a dark stain if left to dry.

Rose Hip Compress

Ingredients:
rose hips, water

Instructions:
1. Add 1 teaspoon rose hips to 1 cup boiling water.
2. Simmer for 2 minutes.
3. Strain, then cool.
4. Dip cotton balls into the solution and apply to eyelids for 10 minutes.

AUTHOR NOTE: REMEMBER TO PATCH TEST. SOME INDIVIDUALS ARE SENSITIVE TO ROSE HIPS.

Tea Compress

Ingredients:
tea bags, water

Instructions:
1. Simmer brand-name tea bags or chamomile tea bags in water for 5 minutes.
2. Cool bags to room temperature, then apply to eyelids.
3. Leave on for 10 minutes while you lie down and prop up your feet.

PROBLEMS AND SOLUTIONS

Crow's Feet Treatment 1

Ingredients:
comfrey, water, lanolin, sunflower oil, egg yolk

Instructions:
1. Add 1 teaspoon comfrey to 1 cup boiling water. Let steep for 5 minutes. Strain and set aside to cool.
2. Melt 1 teaspoon lanolin in 1 tablespoon sunflower oil.
3. Let cool slightly.
4. Stir in 1 beaten egg yolk.
5. Add 1 teaspoon cooled comfrey infusion.
6. Mix well and use around eyes to soften lines. Discard unused portion after four days.

AUTHOR NOTE: USING OIL AROUND THE EYE AREA BOTHERS SOME INDIVIDUALS. IF YOUR EYES BECOME IRRITATED OR SENSITIVE TO LIGHT, DISCONTINUE USE OF THESE PRODUCTS NEAR THE EYES.

Crow's Feet Treatment 2

Ingredients:
cocoa butter or coconut oil

Instructions:
1. Spread the cocoa butter or coconut oil around the eye area to reduce lines.
2. Apply as often as possible.

AUTHOR NOTE: USING OIL AROUND THE EYE AREA BOTHERS SOME INDIVIDUALS. IF YOUR EYES BECOME IRRITATED OR SENSITIVE TO LIGHT, DISCONTINUE USE OF THESE PRODUCTS NEAR THE EYES.

$\mathcal{H}\overline{AIR}$

Long ago, hair was considered the most powerful, beautiful essence of a person. It was combed, styled, and decorated; it was honored in song, poem, and story. From Samson to Rapunzel, hair has held the place of honor for containing not only strength, but power. Some cultures gather strands of hair to cast spells on the owner. Many Native American tribes cut their hair while mourning the loss of a loved one. Our hair is more than a fashion. It is a living part of us.

As with skin, there are different types of hair. Read the following pages to discover the best way to care for your particular type of hair.

OILY HAIR

Wash your hair, according to the following instructions, once a week. If you have to shampoo again, do it midweek or as often as necessary. In between shampoos, you may try brushing your hair with dry cornmeal, oatmeal, or bran to remove oiliness. If using cornmeal, you may want to apply it with rubber gloves, as it will remove the oil from the skin of your hands as well as from your oily scalp. Always use a clean brush with natural bristles, and be sure to comb thoroughly to remove all of the meal.

Follow these instructions for shampooing oily hair:

1. Brush your hair thoroughly, at least 50 strokes.

2. After you brush it, steam it for 10 minutes.
3. Apply a mild shampoo or use a shampoo bar.
4. Rinse and shampoo again.
5. Rinse thoroughly with cool water for at least 1 full minute.
6. Apply Final Rinse (see pages 52–54), tilting your head back to let the water flow from the top of the head down. This makes the hair cuticles close and become smooth and glossy, which allows light to reflect off your hair for a natural shine.
7. Gently towel dry. Do not wring or rub hair.

DRY HAIR

Wash your hair once a week, according to shampooing instructions that follow. It is important to steam your hair, but only necessary to do so once or twice a month. In between shampoos, brush with dry shampoo of oatmeal or cornmeal to keep hair clean. You may want to use rubber gloves to apply the meal or be sure to apply moisturizer to your hands after using it, because it will remove oil from your fingers as well as from your scalp. Take care to brush thoroughly to remove all the meal.

Follow these instructions for shampooing dry hair:

1. Brush your hair thoroughly, at least 50 strokes.
2. Massage olive oil or sunflower oil into your hair.
3. Steam your hair for 10 minutes.
4. Use a mild shampoo with an egg additive.
5. Rinse and shampoo again.

6. Rinse with warm water, not hot, for at least 1 full minute.
7. Use Final Rinse (pages 53–54) tilting your head back to let the water flow from the top of the head down. This closes the hair cuticles and makes them smooth and glossy, which allows light to reflect off your hair for a natural shine.
8. Gently towel dry.

SHAMPOOS

You may use any or all of the following additives. Add them to 8 ounces of your favorite mild shampoo or to the following shampoo recipes.

- ⁊ One whole egg. (Refrigerate the shampoo between uses.)
- ⁊ One tablespoon liquid lecithin.
- ⁊ One tablespoon unflavored gelatin.

Quick Herbal Shampoo for Dark Hair

Ingredients:
dried sage, dried rosemary, dried stinging nettle, water, mild shampoo

Instructions:
1. Add 1 teaspoon dried sage, 1 teaspoon dried rosemary, and 1 teaspoon dried stinging nettle to 1/4 cup boiling water.
2. Turn off heat and steep for 30 minutes.
3. Strain and cool.
4. Mix 2 tablespoons of the herbal infusion into the amount

of mild shampoo you will use during a week's time. Bottle. Refrigerate between uses. Discard unused portion after one week.

5. Add remaining herbal infusion to 1 quart water and use as a final rinse.

Quick Herbal Shampoo for Light Hair

Ingredients:

dried chamomile flowers, dried mullein flowers, water, mild shampoo

Instructions:

1. Add 1 teaspoon dried chamomile flowers and 1 teaspoon dried mullein flowers to 1/4 cup boiling water.
2. Turn off heat and steep for 30 minutes.
3. Strain and cool.
4. Mix 2 tablespoons of the herbal infusion into the amount of mild shampoo you will use during a week's time. Bottle. Refrigerate between uses. Discard unused portion after 1 week.
5. Add remaining herbal infusion to 1 quart water and use as a final rinse.

Herbal Castile Shampoo for Dark Hair

Ingredients:

pure castile soap, water, dried sage leaves, dried rosemary leaves, dried peppermint, peppermint oil, vodka

Instructions:

1. Add 1 tablespoon dried sage leaves, 2 tablespoons dried rosemary leaves, and 1 tablespoon dried peppermint to 2 1/2 cups boiling water (use a glass pot or a glass jar in a pot of water).

2. Reduce heat and simmer for 15 minutes.

3. Cover and steep for 30 minutes.

4. Strain the decoction into another glass pot or a glass jar in a pot of water.

5. Add 2 ounces grated castile soap.

6. Simmer over low heat until soap is completely dissolved, stirring constantly with a wooden spoon.

7. Cool.

8. Mix 2 drops of peppermint oil into 2 tablespoons vodka, then stir this into the shampoo mixture. Whip with hand mixer.

9. Pour into a clean jar and cap it. Let stand in a warm place for a day and shake well before using.

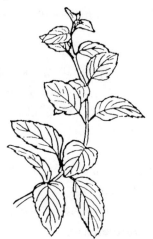

Herbal Castile Shampoo for Light Hair

Ingredients:

pure castile soap, water, dried chamomile flowers, peppermint oil, vodka

Instructions:

1. Add 1/4 cup dried chamomile flowers to 2 1/2 cups boiling water (use a glass pot or a glass jar in a pot of water).
2. Reduce heat and simmer for 15 minutes.
3. Cover and steep for 30 minutes.
4. Strain the decoction into another glass pot or a glass jar in a pot of water.
5. Add 2 ounces grated castile soap.
6. Simmer over low heat until soap is completely dissolved, stirring constantly with a wooden spoon.
7. Cool.
8. Mix 2 drops of peppermint oil into 2 tablespoons vodka, then stir this into the shampoo mixture. Whip with hand mixer.
9. Pour into a clean jar and cap it. Let stand in a warm place for a day and shake well before using.

Shampoo for Dry Hair

Ingredients:

egg whites, water

Instructions:

1. Beat egg whites slightly.
2. Massage egg whites into wet hair and scalp.
3. Rinse hair thoroughly with warm water.

RINSES

Final Rinse for Dark, Oily Hair

This vinegar rinse helps restore the hair's natural acid balance and removes soap, which dulls hair. It also softens the hair and makes it more manageable.

Ingredients:
vinegar, warm water

Instructions:
1. Mix 2 tablespoons apple cider vinegar with 1 quart warm water.
2. Pour through hair, gently squeezing out excess rinse.
3. Towel dry.

Final Rinse for Light, Oily Hair

This rinse is drying and acts as a mild bleach.

Ingredients:
lemon juice, warm water

Instructions:
1. Add 2 tablespoons lemon juice to 1 quart warm water.
2. Pour this rinse through hair after shampooing and rinsing with plain water.
3. Gently squeeze out excess, then towel dry.

Final Rinse: Mint and Rosemary Vinegar

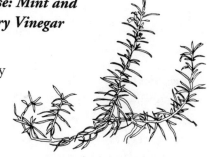

Ingredients:

dried mint, dried rosemary
leaves, dried bergamot or
dried basil or dried sage,
clear apple cider vinegar

Instructions:

1. Put 1/2 tablespoon dried mint, 2 tablespoons dried rosemary leaves, 2 tablespoons dried bergamot, dried basil, or dried sage into a wide-mouthed jar.
2. Heat 1 cup vinegar in a glass pot until it is just about to boil, then pour over the herbs.
3. After the vinegar cools, put two layers of plastic over the jar, then screw on the lid and let it stand in a warm place for one week, shaking it vigorously once a day.
4. Strain herbal vinegar into a bottle. Cap. (If using metal lid, cover inside with plastic so that vinegar is not in contact with metal.)
5. Dilute 1/3 cup of herbal vinegar with 2 cups warm water.
6. Pour this final rinse over hair two or three times, catching it in a bowl each time for reuse.

Final Rinse: Stinging Nettles

NETTLE STRENGTHENS YOUR HAIR. BE SURE TO WEAR GLOVES WHILE GATHERING AND PREPARING STINGING NETTLES FOR SIMMERING.

Ingredients:
stinging nettles, vinegar, water, perfume

Instructions:
1. Put 1/2 cup stinging nettles (1 tablespoon if using dried nettles) with 1/2 cup apple cider vinegar and 1/2 cup water in a jar.
2. Place the jar in a pan of water and simmer for an hour, making sure the pan doesn't boil dry.
3. Strain and cool.
4. Add a few drops of perfume (optional).
5. Pour through your hair, gently squeezing out excess before toweling dry.

CONDITIONERS

Sun, wind, diet, chemicals, color treatment, and styling all contribute to how our hair looks. Too much of any or all of these can be very damaging to our hair, and then we need to take special care to restore it to a healthy state. Even healthy hair can benefit from special conditioning and steaming.

The first three recipes are for general use in conditioning your hair to keep it looking its best. The others are for specific problems.

Body-Adding Conditioner

Ingredients:

dried stinging nettles, water

Instructions:

1. Place 4 tablespoons dried stinging nettles and 1 cup water in a glass jar.
2. Put the glass jar in a pan of water and let this solution simmer for 30 minutes.
3. Strain, cool, then apply to clean hair. Do not rinse out.

Herbal Conditioning Oil

PREPARE ONE WEEK BEFORE USE; STORE IN A GLASS BOTTLE.

Ingredients:

dried chamomile flowers, dried rosemary leaves, sunflower oil

Instructions:

1. Put 1/4 cup dried chamomile flowers, 2 tablespoons rosemary leaves, and 1/2 cup of sunflower oil in a jar.
2. Place jar in a pot of water and heat over moderate flame for 30 minutes.
3. Remove from heat and cover the jar with muslin or cheesecloth, held in place by a rubber band.
4. Let the jar stand in the sun for one week, stirring once a day.
5. At the end of the week, strain through the muslin or cheesecloth into a clean container.
6. Warm the oil over low heat for a few minutes, or warm in microwave. CAUTION: DO NOT OVERHEAT.

7. Wet your hair with hot water, making sure water is not so hot as to burn your scalp, squeezing out excess water.
8. Spread the warm oil through your hair with your fingers.
9. Cover your hair with a shower cap or plastic bag. CAUTION: DO NOT COVER FACE WITH PLASTIC.
10. Soak a heavy hand towel in hot water, wring it out, and wrap it around the plastic covering or shower cap to keep the oil warm. When the towel cools, wet the towel again, taking care not to use water hot enough to burn you. Treat hair for 20 minutes.
11. Shampoo twice, use a final rinse, and towel dry.

Natural Conditioner

Ingredients:
ripe avocado, lemon, finely ground sea salt, aloe

Instructions:
1. Mash 1 ripe avocado and blend with a squeeze of lemon, 1 teaspoon sea salt, and the juice from one leaf of aloe (approximately 1 tablespoon).
2. Comb the mixture through your hair using your fingers.
3. Wrap your hair with plastic. Cover only your scalp area. CAUTION: DO NOT COVER FACE WITH PLASTIC.
4. After 20 to 30 minutes, rinse out the mixture.
5. Shampoo several times to make sure all avocado and aloe residue is out.
6. Use a final rinse and gently towel dry hair.

Sunshine Conditioner

Ingredients:

lemon juice, honey, egg, oil of rosemary, sunflower oil

Instructions:

1. Add 2 teaspoons lemon juice and 1 teaspoon honey to 1 egg.
2. Beat the mixture.
3. Heat the mixture in a double boiler or microwave, stirring constantly. (If using the microwave, stir at 5-second intervals.)
4. When mixture is warm and creamy, remove from the heat and let cool.
5. When it is cool, slowly whisk in 2 drops of oil of rosemary and 1/4 cup sunflower oil.
6. Warm this conditioner and apply to hair 15 minutes before shampooing.

SPECIAL PROBLEMS

Conditioner for Damaged Hair

If your hair has been overstyled or is damaged due to dyeing, bleaching, or perming, try the following remedies:

✿ Mix 2 tablespoons of cider vinegar with 1 quart water. Pour through hair as a final rinse.

✿ Comb a small amount of sunflower oil through your hair and then steam your hair, shampooing after the steam treatment.

✿ After you have applied your night cream or moisturizer (pages 8–11) to your face, clean off your fingertips on the ends of your hair.

❦ Rather than discarding night cream (page 11) that is not used within three weeks, apply it to wet hair and leave on for 30 minutes. Shampoo.

Dandruff Treatment for Dry Hair

Ingredients:
raw linseed oil, cider vinegar, water

Instructions:
1. Rub 2 tablespoons raw linseed oil onto your scalp.
2. Cover your head with a wet hand towel.
3. Sit under a hair drier for half an hour.
4. Remove towel carefully and shampoo your hair.
5. Rinse with mild vinegar and water solution (2 tablespoons vinegar mixed with 1 quart warm water).

Be sure to use raw linseed oil as boiled linseed oil is very sticky to work with. (Boiled linseed oil forms a skin when used to preserve wooden walls. It is often an ingredient in paint.)

AUTHOR NOTE: BE SURE TO PATCH TEST BEFORE USING THIS RECIPE. LINSEED OIL IS SOOTHING TO THE SKIN, UNLESS YOU ARE ALLERGIC.

Dandruff Treatment for Oily Hair 1

Ingredients:
apple cider vinegar, dried mint, water

Instructions:
1. Pour 1/4 cup boiling water over 1 teaspoon dried mint. Let steep for 10 minutes, then strain.

2. Mix the mint infusion with 1/4 cup apple cider vinegar. You may add perfume, if desired.
3. Apply the mixture to your scalp with a cotton ball.
4. Comb, but do not rinse.

Dandruff Treatment for Oily Hair 2

Ingredients:
dried stinging nettles, water

Instructions:
1. Simmer 4 tablespoons dried stinging nettles with 1 cup water for 10 minutes. This may be done in the microwave or in a jar placed in a pan of water.
2. Strain.
3. Cool.
4. Apply to scalp with a cotton ball.
5. Comb, but do not rinse.

Dandruff Treatment for Dark, Oily Hair

Ingredients:
dried rosemary leaves, water, egg white, aloe

Instructions:
1. In a glass jar, mix 2 tablespoons dried rosemary leaves and 1 cup water.
2. Place the glass jar in a pan of water and simmer for 10 minutes (or simmer in microwave).
3. Strain and cool.

4. Add this decoction to 1 beaten egg white and 1 teaspoon aloe.
5. Massage the mixture into your scalp, comb, but do not rinse.

Dandruff Treatment for Light, Oily Hair

Ingredient:

egg white

Instructions:

1. Massage 1 beaten egg white into your scalp.
2. Comb, but do not rinse.

Dry Hair Treatment

Ingredients:

egg yolks, sunflower oil, cider vinegar, water

Instructions:

1. Add 3 egg yolks to 2 tablespoons sunflower oil.
2. Massage solution into hair and leave in for one hour.
3. Shampoo.
4. Rinse with vinegar rinse (2 tablespoons cider vinegar per 1 quart warm water).
5. Towel dry.

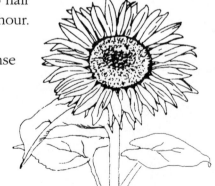

Dull Hair Treatment

Ingredients:
sunflower oil, egg yolks

Instructions:
1. Mix 2 tablespoons sunflower oil with 2 egg yolks.
2. Massage into hair and leave in overnight. Cover your pillow case with a towel and also cover your hair with a bandanna scarf or shower cap.
3. Shampoo thoroughly in the morning.
4. Rinse with cider vinegar solution.

Hair Loss Treatment

The following remedies may be used to help prevent hair from falling out. Remember, as always, that diet is the biggest help. Try eating more protein-rich foods and whole grain cereals. Also remember that heredity plays a big part, and your genes usually win the battle when it comes to hair loss.

Massage any of the following liquids into your scalp before shampooing:

- 🌿 Coconut oil.
- 🌿 Two teaspoons vinegar mixed with 2 tablespoons honey.
- 🌿 One teaspoon rosemary oil simmered for 30 minutes in 8 ounces of water.
- 🌿 One-half cup fresh nettles (gather while wearing gloves) simmered in 1/2 cup water and 1/2 cup vinegar for 30 minutes. Strain and cool before use.

Split Ends Treatment

❧ Use a hairbrush with natural bristles.

❧ Trim the ends every month.

❧ Refer to hair care tips for dry hair and damaged hair.

Restorative and Tonic for Dark Hair 1

Ingredients:

cider vinegar, dried rosemary, dried sage, dried southernwood

Instructions:

1. Place 1 tablespoon of dried rosemary, 1 tablespoon of dried sage, and 1 tablespoon dried southernwood in a jar or glass bottle containing 1 cup vinegar. Cover or cap the bottle. If using a metal lid, cover the jar with plastic first, so that metal is not in contact with vinegar.

2. Place the jar in the sun for a week, shaking every day.

3. Strain.

4. Rub a small amount into your hair and scalp before shampooing.

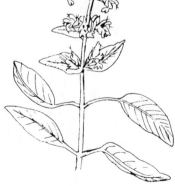

Restorative and Tonic Dark Hair 2

Ingredients:
dried parsley, water

Instructions:
1. Pour 1 cup boiling water over 1 tablespoon dried parsley.
2. Allow to steep for 15 minutes.
3. Strain and cool.
4. Rub this infusion into your hair before shampooing to give shine to dark hair.

Restorative and Tonic for Dry Hair

Ingredients:
sunflower oil, dried sage, dried thyme, dried marjoram, dried balm

Instructions:
1. Place 1 tablespoon dried sage, 1 tablespoon dried thyme, 1 tablespoon dried marjoram, 1 tablespoon dried balm, and 1 cup sunflower oil in a glass bottle or jar. Cover.
2. Allow the oil and herbs to stand in the sun for a week, shaking once a day.
3. Strain.
4. Rub a small amount into your scalp before shampooing.

COLORS, TINTS, AND HIGHLIGHTS

Whatever your hair color, you can intensify the color or highlight it naturally. However, don't expect dramatic color changes like you get with salon mixtures.

The following recipes include directions for adding tints to your shampoo and tinting with rinses. To get the exact color you are looking for takes much experimentation, since factors like the amount of time you let the herbs boil or steep, time of year the herbs are gathered, the potency of the herbs, etc., can alter the results. Remember that the longer you steep herbs, the deeper the color will be. NEVER STEEP HERBS IN ALUMINUM. Always use glass or earthenware. Wash your hair before you tint or highlight it.

Shampoo Additive: Herbal Color Tint for Dark Hair

Simmer 1/2 teaspoon dried sage, 1/2 teaspoon dried nettle, and 1/2 teaspoon dried rosemary in 1/2 cup water for 10 minutes. Strain, cool, and add to 4 ounces of shampoo. Refrigerate. Discard unused portion after 10 days.

Shampoo Additive: Herbal Color Tint for Light Hair

Simmer 2 tablespoons dried chamomile in 1/2 cup water for 10 minutes. Strain, cool, and add to 4 ounces of shampoo. Refrigerate and discard unused portion after 10 days.

Highlighting Rinse for Blonde Hair

Ingredients:

water, dried chamomile flowers, dried mullein flowers, orange blossom water, lemon

Instructions:

1. Bring 2 cups water to a boil in a glass pot, lower heat and stir in 1/2 cup dried chamomile flowers and 2 tablespoons mullein flowers. Simmer for 30 minutes.
2. Cover and steep for 4 hours.
3. Strain.
4. Stir in 1 tablespoon orange blossom water and the juice from 1/2 lemon.
5. Pour the rinse through hair (make sure it's freshly shampooed and rinsed) several times, catching the liquid in a bowl to use again. Do not wash out.
6. Dry your hair in bright sunlight. Use on a regular basis for best results.

Natural Brightening Rinse for Blonde Hair

THIS RINSE RELAXES THE SCALP AND SLOWS DOWN OIL PRODUCTION.

Ingredients:

chamomile tea bags, water

Instructions:

1. Pour 3 quarts boiling water over 10 chamomile tea bags.
2. Let steep for 20 minutes.
3. Remove tea bags and let the infusion cool.

4. Shampoo and condition hair. Rinse.
5. Finally, pour the Natural Brightening Rinse for Blonde Hair over hair again and again, collecting in a bowl each time. Do not wash out.
6. Towel dry hair.

Tint/Rinse for Light Hair

Ingredients:

dried chamomile, water, lemon juice

Instructions:

1. Add 4 tablespoons dried chamomile to 2 cups water and simmer in a glass pot for 30 minutes.
2. Add 1 teaspoon lemon juice.
3. Strain and cool.
4. Rinse through hair several times.
5. Rinse hair with clear water.
6. Towel dry.

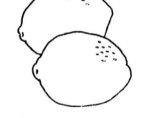

Blonde Tint

USE THIS RECIPE WEEKLY TO BUILD THE COLOR YOU WANT.

Ingredients:

dried chamomile, water, cotton, lemon juice

Instructions:

1. Add a handful (about 1 cup) of dried chamomile flowers to 1 cup water and simmer for 1 hour in a glass pot.

2. Cool the decoction, strain, then apply to the hair with cotton balls.
3. Leave on for 30 minutes, then rinse out with water.
4. Rinse again with lemon juice and water solution (2 tablespoons of lemon juice per 1 quart warm water).

Brown Tint

Ingredients:

dried sage, dried rosemary, water, vinegar, cotton

Instructions:

1. Add a handful of dried sage (about 1 cup) and 1 tablespoon dried rosemary leaves to 1 cup water and simmer for 1 hour in a glass pot.
2. Cool the decoction to room temperature, strain, then apply to wet hair with cotton balls.
3. Leave on for 30 to 60 minutes. The longer you leave it on, the deeper the color will be.
4. Rinse out with water. Rinse again with vinegar and water solution (2 tablespoons apple cider vinegar per 1 quart warm water).

Light Brown Tint

Ingredients:

dried sage, dried rosemary, water, henna, ground cloves, cotton, vinegar

Instructions:

1. Add a handful of dried sage (about 1 cup) and 1 table-spoon dried rosemary to 1 cup water and simmer for 1 hour in a glass pot.
2. Cool the decoction, strain, then add 1 teaspoon henna and 1/2 teaspoon ground cloves to make a thin paste.
3. Work solution into hair and leave in for 30 to 60 minutes, depending on depth of color desired.
4. Rinse with water, then again with vinegar and water solution (2 tablespoons vinegar per 1 quart warm water).

Dark Tint/Rinse

Ingredients:

dried sage, dried rosemary, water, vinegar

Instructions:

1. Add 4 tablespoons dried sage and 2 tablespoons dried rosemary to 2 cups of water. Simmer in a glass pot for 30 minutes.
2. Strain and cool.
3. Rinse through hair several times.
4. Rinse with clear water.
5. As a final rinse, use a vinegar and water solution (2 table-spoons cider vinegar per 1 quart water).

Rinse to Deepen Color of Dark Hair

Ingredients:

water, tea bags, dried sage leaves, dried rosemary leaves

Instructions:

1. Pour 2 cups boiling water over 2 tea bags.
2. Steep, covered, in a glass pot, for 15 minutes.
3. In another bowl or glass pot, mix 1/4 cup dried sage leaves and 3 tablespoons dried rosemary leaves.
4. Remove the tea bags, squeezing out all the liquid.
5. Reheat the tea; pour it over the herbs when it begins to boil.
6. Cover and steep for 1 hour.
7. Strain and cool.
8. Pour the rinse through your freshly shampooed and rinsed hair, catching the liquid in a bowl so that you may rinse several times.

Natural Brightener for Red Hair

BECAUSE OF ITS ACIDITY, THIS RINSE TIGHTENS HAIR CUTICLES, WHICH BOOSTS THE SHINE AND ENHANCES THE RED COLOR TO MAKE IT MORE VIBRANT.

Ingredients:

cranberry juice

Instructions:

1. Saturate hair with cranberry juice.
2. Leave on hair for 2 minutes, then shampoo out with a gentle shampoo.
3. Use an instant conditioner following the shampoo.

Natural Brightening Rinse for Red Hair

THIS RINSE NATURALLY BRIGHTENS GOLD OR RED TONES.

Ingredients:
lemon juice, lime juice, water

Instructions:
1. Mix 1/4 cup lemon juice, 1/4 cup lime juice, and 1/2 cup water.
2. Bottle the mix in a spritzer, then spritz on hair.
3. Sit in the sun for 15 minutes.

Reddish Tint

CAUTION: IF THIS RECIPE IS USED CONTINUOUSLY, IT MAY ACCUMULATE AND GIVE HAIR A BRASSY COLOR.

Ingredients:
henna, water, vinegar

Instructions:
1. Simmer 1/2 ounce henna in 1 quart water for 20 minutes.
2. Cool and strain.
3. Rinse through the hair several times, then rinse out with water.
4. As a final rinse, use vinegar and water solution (2 table-spoons apple cider vinegar per 1 quart warm water).

Tonic to Disguise Gray Hair

THIS TONIC WILL KEEP FOR ONE WEEK IN THE REFRIGERATOR.

Ingredients:
loose tea, dried sage, water

Instructions:
1. Put 1 tablespoon loose tea and 1 tablespoon dried sage into a jar, then pour 2 cups boiling water over the herbs.
2. Place the jar in a pan of water and simmer for 2 hours.
3. Cool and strain.
4. Rub into the scalp every day. Gradually the gray should disappear and your hair will become brown.

AUTHOR NOTE: YOU WILL NEED TO CONTINUE USE OF THIS DECOCTION ONCE YOU START, OR YOUR HAIR MAY TAKE ON A GREENISH TINT.

SETTING LOTIONS AND HAIR SPRAYS

Mousse and Molding Gel

The following may be used to help your hair retain the shape you give it:

- Beat an egg white. Apply with fingertips.
- Make a molding gel of 1 teaspoon unflavored gelatin and 1 tablespoon hot water. Comb through the hair before the gelatin sets up. A little goes a long way, so use sparingly and make sure there are no undissolved clumps left in your hair.

❧ Simmer 4 tablespoons flaxseed in 1 cup water for 30 minutes. Cool, strain, apply.

Flaxseed Setting Lotion

Ingredients:
flaxseed, water

Instructions:
1. Bring 1 cup water to boil in a glass pot, then reduce heat and stir in 4 tablespoons crushed flaxseed.
2. Simmer about 20 minutes, stirring occasionally.
3. Strain and apply to hair with tips of fingers.

Hair Spray

Ingredients:
lemon peel, water, sugar

Instructions:
1. Peel 1 lemon and put the strips of peel in a glass pot containing 2/3 cup water.
2. Boil lemon peels in water until the mixture is slightly sticky (about five minutes at a rolling boil).
3. Strain.
4. Add a pinch of sugar and bottle in a spritz bottle.

AUTHOR NOTE: TREAT YOURSELF TO A LEMONY FACIAL STEAM BY STANDING ABOUT 12 INCHES OVER THE POT WHILE IT BOILS. BE CAREFUL NOT TO BURN YOURSELF.

$\mathcal{L}$IPS, $\mathcal{T}$EETH, AND $\mathcal{M}$OUTH

A smile is one of the most welcome sights in the world, especially when the mouth that smiles shows a set of white teeth. Good dental care is important, as are visits to the dentist. Read the next few pages for natural methods.

LIPS

For cracked or dry lips, soothe them with either lanolin, castor oil, or cocoa butter.

Lip Gloss

Ingredients:
cocoa butter, beeswax, coconut oil, almond oil, aloe, honey, liquid lanolin, vitamin E oil

Instructions:
1. Melt 1 teaspoon grated cocoa butter, 1/4 teaspoon grated beeswax, 1/2 teaspoon coconut oil, and 1/2 teaspoon almond oil in a glass beaker in the microwave, stirring at 10-second intervals.
2. Quickly whisk in 1/4 teaspoon honey, 1/4 teaspoon aloe, a few drops of liquid lanolin, and a few drops of vitamin E oil.
3. Pour into a small container (a contact lens case works well). Stir once more before it solidifies.

TEETH

The best possible way to keep your teeth healthy is to eat an apple every day and to eat foods high in calcium.

Natural tooth cleansers for brushing can be made easily. Here are a few ideas:

- ❦ Use baking soda on a wet toothbrush.
- ❦ Brush your teeth and gums with saltwater.
- ❦ Rub a leaf of sage over your teeth to keep them white.
- ❦ Eat raspberries to help dissolve tartar on your teeth.
- ❦ Lakota tribes used juice from wild strawberries to cleanse their teeth and gums. The juice was supposed to aid in fastening loose teeth, keeping the teeth white, and preventing gums from becoming foul.

Herbal Tooth Powder

Ingredients:
dried shavegrass, dried white oak bark, dried oat straw, dried comfrey root, dried peppermint, cloves

Instructions:
1. Combine 1 teaspoon each of the listed herbs.
2. Grind to a fine powder.
3. Place in a small container.
4. To use, sprinkle the powder over your wet toothbrush.

Mouthwashes

Natural mouthwashes are very effective. If you have bad breath, try the following:

- ❧ Chew a little fresh parsley.
- ❧ Rinse your mouth with water containing chopped watercress.
- ❧ Rinse your mouth with apple juice.
- ❧ Rinse your mouth with salt water (1/2 teaspoon salt in 1 cup water).
- ❧ A fresh leaf of spearmint helps whiten the teeth, condition the gums, and also prevents bad breath.

Herbal Mouthwash

Ingredients:
dried balm, dried savory, dried thyme

Instructions:

1. Combine 1 teaspoon each of dried balm, dried savory, and dried thyme.
2. Pour 1 cup boiling water over the herbs.
3. Cool and strain into a clean bottle.
4. Rinse out your mouth with a portion of the infusion.
5. Refrigerate the remainder. Discard unused portion after four days.

$\mathcal{H}$ANDS AND $\mathcal{N}$AILS

HANDS

Preventative care is the best when it comes to your hands, just as it is with every other area. Wear gloves when you work outside. Wear rubber gloves to protect hands from harsh house-cleaning agents.

Always smooth your moisturizer or night cream onto your hands as well as on your face and neck.

Treatment for Chapped or Rough Hands 1

Ingredients:
oatmeal, water, lemon juice, olive oil

Instructions:

1. Add 1/4 cup oatmeal to 1/2 cup water and steep for 10 minutes.
2. Add 1 tablespoon lemon juice and 1 teaspoon olive oil.
3. Cool for a few minutes, then rub mixture into hands.
4. Leave on for a few minutes, then rinse off.

AUTHOR NOTE: THIS RECIPE MAKES MORE THAN YOU'LL USE ON YOUR HANDS IN ONE APPLICATION, SO YOU CAN ALSO USE IT ON KNEE CAPS, ELBOWS, AND HEELS A FEW MINUTES BEFORE YOU SHOWER.

Treatment for Chapped or Rough Hands 2

Ingredients:

cocoa butter, almond oil, lanolin, vinegar

Instructions:

1. Heat 1 tablespoon grated cocoa butter, 1 tablespoon almond oil, 1 tablespoon lanolin together until melted.
2. Whisk in 1/2 teaspoon vinegar.
3. Pour into clean wide-mouth jar.
4. Rub mixture into hands.

Treatment for Brown Spots or Discoloration of Hands

Ingredients:

lemon rind or raw potato

Instructions:

1. Rub area of discoloration with the inside of a lemon peel or slice of raw potato. Do not use the peel of the potato, since it may leave a dark stain.
2. Moisturize your hands following this treatment.

NAILS

Nails are part of the epidermal structure, like a thick skin. The function of the nails is to protect the fingers and toes, especially the sense of touch of the fingers. The nails also can tell us about health problems. For a fingernail to reproduce itself, it takes 100 to 150 days; toenails take 300 to 450 days.

Be good to your nails. Never use anything metallic or sharp to clean them. If you wear nail polish, let your nails "breathe" at least once a week.

The following advice is recommended for nails on both the hands and the feet.

Dietary Supplement for Healthy Nails

As with everything else, your nails are affected by your diet. If you lack protein in your diet, your nails may become soft.

Ingredients:
unflavored gelatin, milk, peanut oil, molasses

Instructions:
1. Warm 1 cup milk.
2. Add 1 teaspoon unflavored gelatin, 1/4 teaspoon peanut oil, and 1 teaspoon molasses. If gelatin does not dissolve, microwave for 30 seconds.
3. Drink this three times a day.

Treatment for Brittle or Split Nails

Ingredients:
castor oil, olive oil, lecithin

Instructions:
1. Mix 1/4 teaspoon castor oil, 1/4 teaspoon olive oil, and 1/4 teaspoon liquid lecithin.
2. Rub into nails and around the nail area.

Treatment for Soft Nails

Ingredients:

egg yolk, linseed oil

Instructions:

1. Blend together 1 egg yolk and 1 tablespoon linseed oil.
2. Massage this mixture into your nails.

Cuticle Softener and/or Nail Bleach

Ingredients:

egg yolk, pineapple juice, lemon juice

Instructions:

1. Mix together 1 egg yolk and 1 tablespoon pineapple juice.
2. Add a few drops of lemon juice.
3. Soak nails in this solution for 15 minutes.

Nail Polish

As a substitute for commercial nail polish, try buffing your nails with beeswax or cocoa butter and a soft cloth.

$\mathcal{L}$EGS AND $\mathcal{F}$EET

VARICOSE VEINS

I know from experience that varicose veins can be very painful and really unattractive. My advice for varicose veins is to wear loose-fitting clothing and stockings; follow an exercise program that is not jolting to your legs (swimming and hiking); avoid standing or sitting in the same position for long periods; and elevate your legs whenever possible, especially when pregnant.

Try this exercise for varicose veins:

For best results, place a leg rest (such as a folded blanket) about 8 or 10 inches high at the foot of the bed or couch. Lying flat on the bed (or couch), raise and rest the leg on the leg rest for 15 seconds. Next, lower the leg below the level of the bed (or couch) for 3 minutes.

Repeat the cycle, alternating legs, for half an hour. This exercise is beneficial due to the raising and lowering of the leg, which alternately fills and empties blood vessels of the lower leg.

Other helpful ideas for varicose veins include the following:

- Drink white oak bark tea.
- Take baths in comfrey to improve circulation.
- Pour 1 cup boiling water over 1 tablespoon of yellow dead nettle (*Lamium galeobdolon*). Steep for 15 minutes, then strain. Use the infusion as a compress on your legs.
- Soak your feet with various footbaths (pages 86–88) and then massage them with oils or your moisturizer.

Ointment for Varicose Veins

Ingredients:

marigold (*calendula*) leaves, stems, and flowers; lard; linen

Instructions:

1. Melt 2 cups of lard in a glass pot.
2. Add 4 cups of finely chopped marigold leaves, stems, and flowers.
3. Stir, cover the pot, and remove from the stove. Let stand for one day.
4. The next day, warm the mixture and filter it into clean jars, using muslin, cheesecloth, or linen as a filter.
5. Spread the ointment, thickly, on a piece of linen, and loosely bandage your legs with it. For daily use, spread the ointment into the legs.

FEET

It was first brought to my attention in college that I was a foot-abuser. My roommate could hardly believe that I neglected my feet so. But then, what could one expect from a midwestern farmer's daughter? My southern sister taught me, among other things, the importance of caring for my feet. And I'm glad she did, because shortly thereafter I met a man with a foot fetish who taught me the simple pleasures of going barefoot and enjoying a foot massage.

Thanks, Denisa. And thank you, Jim.

Reflexology: The Art of Foot Massage

Our feet take a lot of daily abuse, because they are under pressure of our body weight. It is believed that by massaging the feet we can bring about relaxation of the entire body. It is also believed that certain areas of the feet correspond with areas of the body (see diagram). Reflexologists massage the feet to reduce stress and induce relaxation. There are thousands of nerves in the feet, so this stimulation opens and clears the neural pathways. Foot massage also improves circulation.

By massaging certain points of your feet, you should be able to relax the corresponding area. For example, if you have a headache, you would massage your toes. The area beneath your big toe can be massaged to alleviate neck tension. To relieve cramps, try massaging the heel area up to the middle of your foot.

There are dozens of articles and books on the subject that you may want to read to learn more about reflexology. For the purposes of this book, I'd like to introduce the idea to you and let you feel the benefits of caring for your feet.

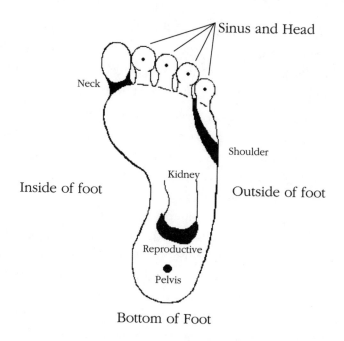

Sinus and Head

Neck

Inside of foot

Kidney

Outside of foot

Shoulder

Reproductive

Pelvis

Bottom of Foot

Simple Reflexology Techniques

Before you begin, soak your feet in warm water or wipe them with a warm, wet washcloth. Rub in a small amount of moisturizer, night cream, or perfumed oil all over both feet. If the cream or oil has not soaked in before you practice the reflexology techniques, wipe your feet with a towel. Practice all the techniques on one foot before moving to the other, starting with the left foot. The most comfortable position to perform these techniques may be sitting cross-legged on the floor.

The hardest part of the routine is remembering it. Since it may be awkward to keep the book in front of you each time you do the exercises, try and associate each step with a phrase. I associate the steps with Cinderella at the ball (in italics).

1. Grasp foot with corresponding hand (left hand grabs left foot) with your thumb on the arch and your fingers on top of the foot. Use your little finger to hold the ankle steady. With the other hand, swivel upper foot gently back and forth. *Swivel 'round the ball*

2. Next, work on the big toe. Cup all toes in palm of hand and rub your big toe with your thumb and first finger, using a rhythmic back-and-forth motion. Continue on the other toes, working your way down to the little toe. *Dance on your toes*

3. Place your thumb across the base of your toes and the rest of your hand on the top of your foot, so that you have a good grasp on your upper foot. Now make a fist with the other hand. Press your fist, using the backs of your fingers—not the knuckles—into the ball of your foot. Alternate pressing and squeezing your foot with the hand holding the foot. *Masquerade ball*

4. Grasp the base of each toe, firmly but gently, between the thumb and index finger. Stretch it by stretching the toe gently away from the base. Next, rotate the toe clockwise then counterclockwise. Do this to all your toes. *Twirl to and fro*

5. Prop up your foot. Place your hands on either side of your foot, then lightly pass the foot back and forth between your hands. *Clock strikes twelve, so pass them all by*

6. With a feather touch, repeatedly run your fingertips down the top, bottom, and sides of your foot, moving from ankle to toes. *With a feathery touch, it's time to fly*

FOOT CARE

Athlete's Foot Treatment

Ingredients:
hot water, thyme oil, olive oil, cloves

Instructions:
1. The day before you want to soak your feet, add 12 cloves to 1 teaspoon olive oil. Let sit for 24 hours.
2. Pour 1 gallon hot water in a footbath or a plastic dishpan large enough to accommodate your feet.
3. Add 2 drops of thyme oil.
4. Strain clove/olive oil into footbath.
5. Soak your feet for 15 to 30 minutes, adding hot water as necessary.
6. Towel dry, taking care to dry thoroughly between toes.

Calluses and Rough Feet

For calluses and rough feet, you may use a pumice stone after your footbath to massage away rough skin. After soaking the feet for a few minutes, wet the pumice stone and rub your wet skin area in a circular motion with light-to-medium pressure. To gradually remove built-up calluses, use the stone daily.

Native Americans used to scour their feet with the base of the root of yucca to keep feet smooth and soft.

For rough feet, be sure to soak them and use the night cream or moisturizer on them once a week or more.

Corns

Ingredients:
roasted onion, soft soap

Instructions:
1. Dip one piece of roasted onion in soft soap (pages 105–106).
2. Apply this mixture to the corn on a piece of linen, as a poultice.

AUTHOR NOTE: TO PREVENT CORNS, WEAR SHOES THAT FIT AND PAY CLOSE ATTENTION TO YOUR FEET.

Foot Odor

Make a foot powder of 1/4 cup arrowroot powder and 1/4 cup marigold flowers (*calendula*) to help prevent foot odor. Or sprinkle baking soda over your toes.

FOOTBATHS

A real treat after a day of being on your feet is to pamper yourself with a footbath.

You can soak your feet in a variety of herbs for different results. The main thing to remember is whether you want to stimulate your nerves or soothe them. (See the appendix and also the section on baths for suggestions on relaxing or stimulating herbs.) If you are soaking your feet to prepare for an evening out, try a stimulating footbath. If you want to relax before you sleep, try herbs that soothe. I have had a few sleepless nights because I made the mistake of soaking my feet in lavender or mint before bedtime.

Alfalfa and Mint Footbath

Ingredients:
hot water, sea salt, dried alfalfa, dried mint

Instructions:
1. Pour 1 gallon hot water into a footbath or a plastic dish-pan large enough to accommodate your feet.
2. Add 2 tablespoons sea salt, 2 tablespoons dried alfalfa, and 1 tablespoon dried mint. If you have ticklish or sensitive feet, put the herbs in a tea ball or muslin bag before adding to the hot water.
3. Soak your feet for about 20 minutes, adding more hot water as necessary.
4. Dry feet thoroughly, taking care to dry between your toes.
5. Massage lotion, moisturizer, night cream, or perfumed oil into your feet and follow with the reflexology techniques.

Thyme for a Footbath

Thyme helps soothe your nerves.

Ingredients:
hot water, dried thyme, olive oil

Instructions:

1. Pour 1 cup hot water over 1 tablespoon dried thyme. Let steep for 15 minutes, then strain.
2. Pour 1 gallon hot water into a footbath or a plastic dish-pan large enough to accommodate your feet.
3. Add the infusion of thyme and 1 tablespoon olive oil.
4. Soak your feet about 20 minutes, adding more hot water as necessary.
5. Dry feet thoroughly, taking care to dry between your toes.
6. Massage lotion, moisturizer, night cream, or perfumed oil into your feet and follow with the reflexology techniques.

Eucalyptus Footbath for Tired, Sore Feet

Ingredients:

hot water, dried eucalyptus

Instructions:

1. Pour 1 cup hot water over 1 tablespoon dried eucalyptus. Let steep for 15 minutes, then strain.
2. Pour 1 gallon hot water into your footbath or a plastic dish pan large enough to accommodate your feet.
3. Add the infusion of eucalyptus.
4. Soak your feet about 20 minutes, adding more hot water as necessary.
5. Dry feet thoroughly, taking care to dry between your toes.
6. Massage chamomile lotion (page 100) into your feet and follow with the reflexology techniques.

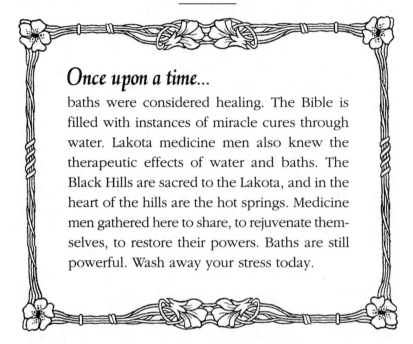

Once upon a time...

baths were considered healing. The Bible is filled with instances of miracle cures through water. Lakota medicine men also knew the therapeutic effects of water and baths. The Black Hills are sacred to the Lakota, and in the heart of the hills are the hot springs. Medicine men gathered here to share, to rejuvenate themselves, to restore their powers. Baths are still powerful. Wash away your stress today.

There is nothing more rejuvenating than a bath, especially if you add salts or herbs to enhance the water's natural restorative powers. The water should be about body temperature (98 degrees Fahrenheit). Hot baths (over 104 degrees Fahrenheit) do more harm than good, especially if you are pregnant or have diabetes, so keep it cool to warm. Don't spend more than half an hour in the tub, or your skin will become dry (prune effect).

The following suggestions are for herbal baths. The herbs can be used alone or mixed. See the appendix for suggested bath herbs, and experiment until you find a combination you really like.

The rule of thumb for herbal baths is to add a strong infusion, or tea, to your bath water; or use a muslin or cheese-cloth bag directly in your bath.

HERBS

Crush the herbs slightly to release their fragrance, mixing them with your hands at the same time. Once you have se-lected and crushed the herbs, select a method for adding the herbs to your bath. Here are three:

1. If you don't have a muslin bag, you can make one by placing the herbs in the center of a piece of muslin (9 inches square), bringing the edges together to form a sack around the mixture. Secure the ends with a string or rubber band and hang the bag from the tub faucet, allowing the hot water to flow through it. After the tub is full, drop the bag in the water and let it steep for 5 minutes or until the tub is cool enough to enter. (This also works well with a mesh tea ball.)

2. Wrap a handful of herbs in cheesecloth. Steep in boiling wa-ter for 15 minutes, then add the tea and wrapped herbs to your bath.

3. Make an infusion by pouring 1 quart boiling water over 1 cup herbs. Allow the herbs to steep for 15 minutes. Strain and pour the infusion into your bath water.

STIMULATING HERBAL BATHS

These baths are not recommended before bedtime.

For a stimulating bath, try adding oil of spearmint or floating a few fresh sprigs of mint in hot bath water. Fresh or dried flowers or leaves of lavender infused in your bath leaves you fragrant. Other herbs that are members of the stimulating mint family are basil, marjoram, rosemary, sage, savory, and thyme.

A bunch of salad burnet tied in cheesecloth or muslin and used in a hot bath can be refreshing and invigorating. Bay, fennel, and marigold flowers are also stimulating herbs. Lovage is a stimulating as well as a deodorizing herb. A strong tea made from the leaves of lovage can be added to a hot bath after a workout.

Stimulating Herbal Bath 1

Ingredients:

dried rosemary, dried lavender, dried mint, cider vinegar

Instructions:

1. Pour 1 cup boiling vinegar over 1/2 tablespoon dried rosemary, 1/2 tablespoon dried lavender, and 1/2 teaspoon dried mint.
2. Let steep for one hour. Strain.
3. Add to bath water.

Stimulating Herbal Bath 2

Ingredients:
dried basil, dried eucalyptus,
dried peppermint

Instructions:
1. Place 1 teaspoon basil,
1 teaspoon eucalyptus, and
1 teaspoon peppermint in a
muslin bag.
2. Run hot water over the bag in your tub and let steep until
water has cooled enough to allow you to soak comfortably.

Relaxing Herbal Baths

These baths are recommended to induce sleep.

For relaxation and fragrance, nothing beats fresh or dried
angelica leaves in your bath. Balm both cleanses and perfumes the skin. Chamomile, comfrey, elder flowers, linden
flowers, and mullein flowers all make relaxing herbal baths.

Sweet, Fragrant Relaxing Bath

Ingredients:
dried chamomile, dried elder flowers, dried linden flowers,
dried lavender flowers, dried angelica, freshly cut rose,
fresh rose geranium petals

Instructions:
1. Put 1 teaspoon dried chamomile, 1 teaspoon dried elder
flowers, 1 teaspoon dried linden flowers, 1 teaspoon dried

lavender flowers, and 1 teaspoon dried angelica into cheesecloth or muslin bag.
2. Place the bag under hot running water in your tub.
3. Let steep until water is cooled to desired temperature.
4. As you climb in to soak, float one cut rose and a few fresh rose geranium petals in your bathwater.

Tonic Citrus Bath

Ingredients:

dried alfalfa, dried comfrey, dried parsley, fresh lemon peel, fresh orange peel

Instructions:

1. Put 1 teaspoon dried alfalfa, 1 teaspoon dried comfrey, 1 teaspoon dried parsley, part of a peel from one lemon and part of peel from one orange into cheesecloth or muslin bag.
2. Place the bag under hot running water in your tub.
3. Let steep until water is cooled to desired temperature.

OILS

Add 2 tablespoons avocado, almond, or sesame oil and 2 or 3 drops perfume or herbal essential oils to your tub.

For increased effectiveness, soak for five minutes first, then add oil to seal in the moisture your body has absorbed from the water.

CAUTION: GET IN AND OUT OF THE TUB CAREFULLY, AS THE OIL WILL MAKE THE TUB SLIPPERY.

Bubble Bath

Ingredients:

safflower oil, shampoo

Instructions:

1. Mix together 4 tablespoons safflower oil and 1 tablespoon of your favorite shampoo.
2. Pour into running bath water.

Stimulating Herbal Bath Oil

Ingredients:

almond oil, bergamot oil, thyme oil, clove oil, lavender oil, eucalyptus oil, vodka

Instructions:

1. Mix together 4 tablespoons almond oil, 2 drops bergamot oil, 2 drops thyme oil, 2 drops clove oil, 2 drops lavender oil, 2 drops eucalyptus oil, and 1 tablespoon vodka.
2. Put in a jar that seals tightly.
3. Shake well every day for one week.
4. Add 1 teaspoon to your bathwater after you have soaked for a few minutes.

SALTS AND MORE

Bath to Relieve Itching 1

Ingredients:

apple cider vinegar

Instructions:
1. Add 1 cup apple cider vinegar to a tepid bath.
2. Soak for 10 minutes.

Bath to Relieve Itching 2

Ingredients:
  cornstarch, hot water

Instructions:
1. Add 1/2 to 1 pound cornstarch to 1 gallon very hot water.
2. Add this solution to tub of warm water (about 98 degrees Fahrenheit).
3. Soak for 15 minutes.

Lavender Meal Bath

Ingredients:
  oatmeal, lavender flowers

Instructions:
1. Mix 1/3 cup oatmeal with 1 tablespoon lavender.
2. Place in a muslin or cotton bath bag.
3. Place bag under hot running water and let it soak a few minutes before bathing.
4. You may use the bag as a scrub cloth while you bathe to smooth, soften, and perfume your skin.

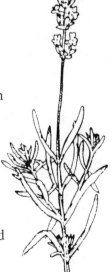

Oatmeal and Bran Bath

Ingredients:
oatmeal, bran, almond meal

Instructions:
1. Mix 1/2 cup oatmeal, 1 cup bran, and 4 tablespoons almond meal.
2. Place in a muslin or cotton bath bag.
3. Place bag under hot running water and let it soak a few minutes before bathing.
4. You may use the bag as a scrub cloth while you bathe.

Bath Salts

Ingredients:
soft soap, food coloring, coarse sea salt

Instructions:
1. Heat 3 ounces soft soap (see pages 105–106 for the soft soap recipe) in the microwave or in the top of a double boiler. If the soft soap is not colored, add food coloring at this point.
2. Put 2 cups coarse sea salt in a large mixing bowl. Pour heated soft soap over the salt.
3. Stir continuously while the mixture cools.
4. Spread the salts out in a thin layer on a cookie sheet and pat them dry with paper towels.
5. Put the bath salts into a decorative container when they are completely dry.
6. Add a handful to the tub under hot running water.

After-Bath Rinse

If you use soap in your bath, rinse off with a mild vinegar and water solution. This helps close the pores after a hot bath.

Apply a body lotion or body oils while you are still damp, to lock in moisture and leave your skin feeling silky soft.

LOTIONS

Once upon a time...

the Greeks used oils to cleanse themelves. They saturated their bodies with oil, then scraped it off. Dead skin and dirt came off with the oil, leaving them clean and with a thin layer of oil for absorption. Native Americans used bear grease in a similar fashion, rubbing their skin with the root of a yucca to soften it.

The skin needs to be cared for and kept moist so it stays smooth and supple.

Body Rubs

* Alternate layers of fresh basil leaves, coarse sea salt, and safflower oil in a jar. Seal. After one week, strain and use the oil as a toning body rub.
* Rather than discarding old perfume bottles, fill them with almond oil. Enough scent lingers to make a fragrant oil that can be used for a delightful body massage.

Rose and Glycerin Gel

Ingredients:

gelatin, water, rose water, glycerin

Instructions:

1. Mix together 1 teaspoon rose water and 3 tablespoons glycerin.
2. In a separate bowl, dissolve 1 teaspoon plain gelatin in 1/2 cup hot water.
3. Blend and pour into a clean jar.

Rose Water and Glycerin Lotion

Ingredients:

rose oil, distilled water, glycerin

Instructions:

1. Add 1/2 teaspoon of soluble rose oil to 1/4 cup distilled water to make rosewater. Or, bruise a handful of petals and gently warm them in 1/4 cup water. Let them steep overnight, then strain off the fragrant water.
2. Make the appropriate strength lotion for your skin type: 1/4 cup rose water and 1 and 1/2 tablespoons glycerin (normal skin); 1/4 cup rose water and 3/4 tablespoon glycerin (oily skin); 1/4 cup rose water and 1/4 tablespoon glycerin (dry skin).
3. Blend rose water with the glycerin until you have a smooth, creamy mixture.
4. Pour into a clean bottle and cap.

Chamomile Lotion

THIS LOTION IS GOOD FOR SUNBURN AND ALSO FOR ACHING FEET.

Ingredients:
chamomile tea bag, water, glycerin

Instructions:
1. Pour 1 cup boiling water over 1 chamomile tea bag.
2. Let steep for 5 minutes, then remove the bag, taking care to squeeze out all the liquid.
3. Cool.
4. Add this infusion to 1/4 cup glycerin.
5. Bottle.
6. Shake well before applying.

Insect Lotion

Ingredients:
dried chamomile, dried nettle, water, cedar needle essence, vinegar

Instructions:
1. Simmer 1 teaspoon dried chamomile and 1 teaspoon dried nettle in 1/2 cup water for 15 minutes. (Use a glass pot or a glass jar in a pot of water.)
2. Strain and cool.
3. Add a few drops of cedar needle essence and 1/4 teaspoon vinegar.
4. Pour in a plastic spritz bottle (vinegar reacts with metal). Refrigerate.

5. Shake well before spritzing on skin. Discard unused portion after 10 days.

Sun Lotion

There are many sunscreens on the market today that offer protection from the sun, but for ultimate protection, wear hats and clothing that do not allow exposure to our skin's worst enemy. That is how our pioneer foremothers did. They also used a recipe similar to this one to prevent sunburn:

Ingredients:
lanolin, peanut oil, apple cider vinegar
Instructions:
1. Melt 1 tablespoon lanolin.
2. Add 1 tablespoon peanut oil. Stir well.
3. Stir in tablespoon apple cider vinegar.
4. Smooth into skin before going out in the sun and then on return from being in the sun.

SOAPS

You can make your own bath soaps by heating soap pieces, adding ingredients, and then molding them. You may use almost any container for a soap mold, such as food molds, butter molds, or candle molds, or you can recycle small plastic containers (yogurt containers work well). If you want to add a little color, just blend in a few drops of candlemaking dye into the melted mixture.

Astringent Soap

Ingredients:

castile soap, water, clove oil, thyme oil, honey, lemon juice, glycerin

Instructions:

1. Grease the molds with petroleum jelly.
2. Place 2 ounces grated soap in a heavy glass pot. Melt over low heat, adding just enough water (up to 1/4 cup) to prevent a film from forming on the pan.
3. When the soap is dissolved and smooth, remove from the heat. If it is clumping, the burner flame is probably too high.
4. Cool slightly, stirring to keep it smooth. Add 2 drops clove oil, 2 drops thyme oil, 2 teaspoons honey, 1 teaspoon lemon juice, and 1 teaspoon glycerin.
5. Pour in the molds.
6. Allow molds to cool overnight in the refrigerator.

7. When you are ready to unmold, dip the mold into hot water or run hot water over the bottom of the container to melt the outside layer of soap, invert the mold over a plate, and tap out the soap.

Meal and Lavender Scrub Soap

Ingredients:

dried lavender, water, castile soap, uncooked oatmeal (you may substitute almond meal or bran)

Instructions:

1. Grease a small yogurt container with petroleum jelly. If you don't have petroleum jelly, use a Styrofoam cup, which will peel off the soap.
2. Make a lavender infusion by adding 2 teaspoons dried lavender to 1/2 cup boiling water. Let steep for 15 minutes.
3. Place 2 ounces grated castile soap in a heavy glass pot or in a glass jar in a pot of water.
4. Strain lavender infusion into the glass pot containing the grated soap. If the soap clumps up, the lavender infusion was too hot.
5. Melt over low heat.
6. When the soap is dissolved, remove from the heat.
7. Cool slightly, stirring to keep it smooth. Add 1/3 cup uncooked meal.
8. Pour in the mold.
9. Place mold in the refrigerator overnight.

10. When you are ready to unmold, dip the mold into hot water to melt the outside layer of soap, invert the mold over a plate, and tap out the soap. If you have used a Styrofoam cup, peel off the Styrofoam.

Orange Blossom Soap

Ingredients:

bar of castile soap, orange blossom water

Instructions:

1. Grease the molds with petroleum jelly.
2. Grate the soap and place it in a heavy glass pot. Melt over low heat, adding just enough orange blossom water (to make orange blossom water, use 1 teaspoon soluble essential oil to 1/2 cup distilled water) to prevent a film from forming on the pan.
3. When the soap is smooth and has the consistency of whipped cream, remove from the heat.
4. Cool slightly, stirring to keep it smooth.
5. Pour in the molds.
6. Allow molds to cool in the refrigerator for a few hours.
7. When you are ready to unmold, dip the mold into hot water to melt the outside layer of soap, invert the mold over a plate, and tap out the soap.

Rose Soap

Ingredients:

bar of castile soap, rose water, glycerin

Instructions:

1. Grease the molds with petroleum jelly.
2. Grate the soap and place it in a heavy glass pot. Melt over low heat, adding just enough rose water to prevent a film from forming on the pan.
3. When the soap is smooth, remove from the heat.
4. Cool slightly, stirring to keep it smooth. Add 1 teaspoon glycerin.
5. Pour in the molds.
6. Allow molds to cool in the refrigerator overnight.
7. When you are ready to unmold, dip the mold into hot water to melt the outside layer of soap, invert the mold over a plate, and tap out the soap.

Soft Soap

Ingredients:

castile soap, water, perfume or essential oil, food coloring

Instructions:

1. Add 1 ounce grated castile soap to 1/2 cup boiling water (use double boiler or jar in a pot of water).
2. Melt until smooth. If any lumps remain, blend for a few seconds with a whisk or a fork or in a blender. Do not heat any longer than necessary.

3. Add a few drops of perfume or essential oil and food coloring to desired shade.
4. Pour into a pump bottle made for soft soap. Cool before use. Makes about 6 ounces.

Comfrey Soft Soap

Ingredients:

castile soap, water, dried comfrey leaves, green food coloring

Instructions:

1. Add 1 teaspoon dried comfrey leaves to 1/2 cup boiling water. Cover, remove from heat, and let steep for 30 minutes. Strain out the leaves, then put the infusion in the top of a double boiler or in a glass jar in a pot of water.
2. Grate 1 ounce castile soap.
3. Add to boiling comfrey infusion.
4. Melt until smooth. If any lumps remain, blend for a few seconds with a whisk or fork or in a blender. Do not heat any longer than necessary.
5. Add a few drops green food coloring.
6. Pour into a pump bottle made for soft soap. Cool before use. Makes about 6 ounces.

SCRUBS

Deep-Cleaning Scrub

Use this scrub once a week for deep cleaning. A total body buffing speeds up the removal of dead cells and surface debris.

Ingredients:

sea salt, olive oil

Instructions:

1. Combine 1/4 cup sea salt with 1/4 cup warm olive oil.
2. Apply to skin with a washcloth to gently buff skin smooth. Pay special attention to elbows, knees, and heels.
3. Alternate long strokes with circular ones, and be careful around blemishes, warts, moles, and varicose veins.
4. Take a hot shower or bath to rinse the oil and salt from your skin.

Yogurt Scrub

Here is another scrub you can use once a week for deep cleaning. It is especially good for cleansing blemished skin.

Ingredients:

plain yogurt, uncooked oatmeal, cornmeal

Instructions:

1. Blend 2 tablespoons plain yogurt, 1 tablespoon uncooked oatmeal, and 1 tablespoon cornmeal together with a fork.
2. Let the mixture warm to room temperature, then apply the scrub to the skin with a massaging motion.
3. Wash thoroughly after use.

Scents

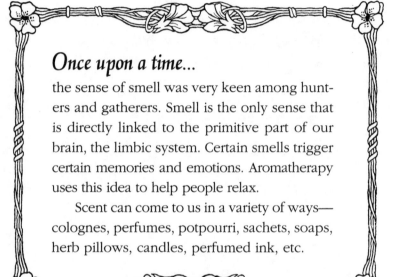

Once upon a time...

the sense of smell was very keen among hunters and gatherers. Smell is the only sense that is directly linked to the primitive part of our brain, the limbic system. Certain smells trigger certain memories and emotions. Aromatherapy uses this idea to help people relax.

Scent can come to us in a variety of ways—colognes, perfumes, potpourri, sachets, soaps, herb pillows, candles, perfumed ink, etc.

Cologne

Here are two suggestions for making your own cologne. Rubbing alcohol dries the skin, so you can use vodka instead, if desired.

- ❦ Combine 1 ounce of an essential oil with 1/4 cup vodka or rubbing alcohol.

❧ Make whatever scent you desire by adding a portion of the substance to an equal amount of vodka or rubbing alcohol and letting it steep. Drain off the liquid each day and add fresh pieces. Do this for several days, until you are satisfied with the scent.

Perfume

All scents begin with some basics. To create your own perfume, try ordering some essential oils and mixing them to your liking. (Start with a few drops at a time to experiment.) Let the mixtures blend for several weeks.

Next, combine a few drops of your favorite essential oil or blend with a few drops of oil (almond oil works well).

$\mathcal{P}$OTPOURRI AND $\mathcal{M}$ORE

Potpourri and sachets really don't have much to do with cosmetics, but adding fragrance to your life certainly makes you feel more lovely and happy by evoking pleasant emotions. I hope you enjoy these recipes.

These dried herbs are very popular in potpourri: angelica leaves, bay leaves, flowers and leaves of bergamot, whole leaves of lemon balm, lavender leaves and flowers, marjoram leaves, flowers and leaves of rosemary.

You may place your potpourri mixture in any decorative container except plastic or aluminum. Warmth helps draw the fragrance. Also, shaking the container will release the perfume. To give new vitality to the mix, you may add extra dried flowers, leaves, and a few drops of essential oil.

Potpourri makes a wonderful gift, too. Once, when I was in the hospital, a friend brought me a basket of the fragrant mixture. The basket came home with me and years later is a reminder of her care and friendship. Thank you, Ruth.

Good Night Potpourri

Ingredients:
2 cups dried rosemary flowers and leaves (prevents bad dreams)

2 cups dried lavender flowers (dissipates melancholy)

1 cup dried thyme (prevents nightmares)

1 cup dried chamomile flowers (soothes nerves)

2 tablespoons dried marjoram (acts as a sedative; it's
   believed to make you dream of your future spouse)
1/2 tablespoon aniseed (fragrant aroma)
1/2 tablespoon powdered orrisroot (fixative)
6 drops bergamot oil
(Optional: lemon verbena leaves, colored petals, or
linden flowers for filler)

Instructions:

1. In a large glass bowl, mix together dried flowers and leaves.
   Set aside.
2. In a small bowl, mix together anise seed, orrisroot, and
   bergamot oil.
3. Add the mixture in the small bowl to the dried flowers
   and leaves.
4. Gently mix with hands.
5. Place this mix in a bowl in your bedroom or tuck a small
   muslin bag filled with this mix in your pillow at night. The
   heat from your body will help release the aromas that will
   help you sleep.

AUTHOR'S NOTE: THIS IS NOT RECOMMENDED FOR PEOPLE WITH ALLER-
GIES OR HAY FEVER.

Lavender Potpourri

Ingredients:

dried lavender flowers, dried marjoram leaves, dried thyme
leaves, dried mint leaves, orrisroot powder, ground
coriander, ground cloves, lavender oil

Instructions:

1. In a large bowl, mix together 1 cup dried lavender flowers, 1/2 cup marjoram leaves, 1 tablespoon dried thyme leaves, and 1 tablespoon dried mint leaves.

2. In a small bowl, blend together 1 tablespoon orrisroot powder, 2 teaspoons ground coriander, and 1/4 teaspoon ground cloves. Stir in a few drops of lavender oil.

3. Add the mixture in the small bowl to the dried flowers and leaves.

4. After mixing well with your hands, you may scoop the potpourri into bowls, baskets, or sachets.

Lover's Potpourri

Ingredients:

2 cups dried peony petals (aphrodisiac)

1 cup dried rosebuds (flowers symbolizing love)

1/2 cup dried jasmine flowers (fragrant)

1 cup dried chamomile flowers (soothes the nerves, symbolizes sound judgment and determination)

1 cup dried linden flowers (relaxing)

1/4 cup dried forget-me-not flowers (sentimental, true love)

1/4 cup dried southernwood (lover's plant)

1/4 cup lemon balm (communication between lovers)

1/4 cup dried basil leaves (love/hate relationship)

1 tablespoon allspice (fragrance)

4 to 5 drops patchouli oil (Do not use much more than this; too much is overpowering.)

Instructions:

1. In a large glass bowl, mix together dried flowers and leaves. Set aside.
2. In a small bowl, blend together patchouli oil with allspice.
3. Add the mixture in the small bowl to the dried flowers and leaves.
4. Gently mix with hands.
5. Store in an empty, clean, wide-mouthed wine bottle (Paul Masson makes these) and cap.
6. To use, pour into two wineglasses and set on the bed stand.

Spicy Floral Potpourri

Ingredients:

dried rose petals, dried geranium leaves, dried lavender leaves and flowers, dried lemon verbena leaves, whole cloves, ground cloves, cinnamon bark, orrisroot powder, ground cinnamon, rose geranium oil, lavender oil

Instructions:

1. In a large glass bowl, mix together 4 cups dried rose petals, 2 cups dried geranium leaves, 2 cups dried lavender leaves and flowers, 1 cup dried lemon verbena leaves, 12 whole cloves, and several pieces of cinnamon bark. Set aside.
2. In a small bowl, blend together 1 teaspoon ground cloves, 2 tablespoons orrisroot powder, and 1 tablespoon ground cinnamon. Add 1 teaspoon rose geranium oil and 1 teaspoon lavender oil, combining them with the powder.

3. Add the mixture in the small bowl to the dried flowers and leaves.

4. After mixing well with your hands, seal the mix in a glass container for one month. After that time, you may scoop the potpourri into bowls, baskets, or sachets.

Fragrant Herb Pillow

An herb pillow uses the warmth of the head to release various aromas which induce relaxation. The following herbs can be substituted for those in the following herb pillow recipe: dried angelica leaves, dried whole leaves of lemon balm, dried bay leaves, dried chamomile flowers, dried hops, and dried marjoram leaves.

Ingredients:

1 cup dried rose petals

1 cup dried lavender flowers

1 cup dried lemon verbena leaves

1 cup dried rosemary leaves and flowers

1 cup dried carnation petals

1 cup dried honeysuckle

1 cup dried lily-of-the-valley

1 cup dried jasmine

ground citrus peel from 2 lemons (fixative)

ground citrus peel from 2 oranges (fixative)

(alternative fixatives are one of the following: 2 teaspoons powdered orrisroot, 2 teaspoons sweet flag root, or 3 drops of oil of bergamot)

Instructions:

1. In a large glass bowl, gently mix together all ingredients with your hands.
2. Place the mix in a decorative pillow, sew shut. The heat from your body will release the aroma.

Rose Bead Necklace

Ingredients:

rose petals, rose oil, unscented vegetable oil

Instructions:

1. Gather fresh rose petals. A quart jar packed full will make a few small beads.
2. Grind the petals in a meat grinder and catch in a glass bowl.
3. Leave standing overnight, uncovered.
4. Repeat for 3 more days, grinding a total of 4 times.
5. After the fourth grinding, rub your hands with unscented vegetable oil, then roll paste between palms to form beads twice the size you want.
6. Stick a pin through the center and stick the bead to a cork board to dry for four days.
7. String the beads, then polish them with rose oil and a damp cloth.

AUTHOR NOTE: DON'T LET THE SUBSTANCE GET TOO DRY, OR IT WON'T STICK TOGETHER TO FORM A BEAD. IF IT STARTS DRYING OUT ON THE THIRD DAY, MAKE THE BEADS THEN. THE SUBSTANCE RESEMBLES HORSE MANURE, BUT SMELLS MUCH BETTER.

Sachet

Pick flowers from your garden, wild herbs from the woods, or whatever you desire, and then dry your pickings. Crush or powder the dried pickings, then add a drop of essential oil to moisturize them. Sew up the mixture into a small, pretty bag and enjoy.

Aroma-Doh

Kids and adults both like "aroma-doh." You can color it any shade and shape it into roses, animals, cars, or just enjoy squeezing it in your hands.

Playing with it reduces stress, especially when herbal oils are added. When your hands work with it and warm it, the scent is released.

CAUTION: DO NOT USE JUST ANY ESSENTIAL OIL IN THIS RECIPE, BECAUSE SOME ARE HIGHLY TOXIC IF INGESTED. REMEMBER THAT SMALL CHILDREN FIND THE AROMA-DOH VERY ATTRACTIVE AND ARE LIKELY TO PUT IT IN THEIR MOUTHS. I SUGGEST ROSE OIL AND THYME OIL, BECAUSE THERE IS NO KNOWN TOXICITY, BUT REMEMBER TO PATCH TEST IN CASE YOU ARE ALLERGIC.

Ingredients:

flour, salt, cream of tartar, water, avocado oil, four different food colorings (use the paste made for coloring cake frosting for brightest colors and best results), rose oil, thyme oil

Instructions:

1. Mix together 2 cups flour, 1 cup salt, and 1 tablespoon cream of tartar.
2. Add 2 cups boiling water. Mix well.
3. When cooled to a comfortable temperature, use hands to mix in 1 tablespoon avocado oil.
4. Divide into 4 equal parts, then add food colorings, mixing well, until the desired shades are achieved. Wash hands between mixing colors and fragrances. Recommended color for thyme aroma-doh is green. Recommended colors for rose aroma-doh are pink, red, or yellow.
5. Add essential oil one drop at a time, mixing well with hands, until the desired aroma is achieved. You can always add oil to renew the aroma.
6. Store in plastic wrap or a covered dish between use.
7. Have fun!

$\mathcal{A}$PPENDIX $\mathcal{A}$: O$_{ILS}$

Each individual has her own skin type. Some people have dry skin, some oily, some a mixture of the two. Choose the oil that suits your skin, your sense of smell, and the type of preparation you are making. The following oils are often used cosmetically:

TYPE	USE	COMMENTS
Almond	hair preparations, nail whitener, eye cream, bath oil	Can cause rash, stuffy nose if allergic; may go rancid
Avocado	hair preparations, face cream, facial mask, bath oil	Good for dry skin
Castor	bath oil, facial mask, lotion	Soothing to the skin
Cocoa Butter	lipstick, soap, lotion, nail preparations	Softens skin; whitens nails; some individuals may be allergic
Coconut	Moisturizer, shampoo, cleanser, hair prepartions, face cream	Some individuals may be allergic
Corn	hair preparations, face cream	Some individuals may be allergic
Lanolin	moisturizer, hair preparations, lip gloss	Made from oil in sheep wool; locks in moisture on skin; some individuals may be allergic

TYPE	*USE*	*COMMENTS*
Linseed	soap, moisturizer, hair preparations	Extracted from flaxseed; some individuals may be allergic
Olive	hair preparations, eyelashes, lips, massage	Penetrates well; some individuals may be allergic
Peanut	hair preparations, nails, ointments, moisturizer, sunburn preparation	Good substitute for almond and olive oils
Safflower	moisturizer, bath oil	Softens the skin; high in polyunsaturates, so it is a light oil good for oily complexions
Sesame	moisturizer, hair preparations	Softens the skin; may help act against lice; may cause rash if allergic
Soybean	bath oil	If allergic, may cause skin eruptions and may also damage hair
Sunflower	hair preparations, facial masks	Contains vitamin E

Appendix B: Herbs

Most preparations you make yourself will not keep as long as cosmetics purchased from the store. Any type of facial, shampoo, rinse, or other recipe containing herbs should be discarded if not used up after four days. Always use utensils and containers that are thoroughly clean when making your beauty preparations, and never mix or store any preparations in aluminum containers.

If you gather your own herbs, there are a few things to remember. Always use caution. Make sure you know what you are gathering and ALWAYS do a patch test on your skin, in case you have made a mistake in plant identification or are allergic to a particular herb or herbal combination.

Also remember that herbs vary in potency according to the type of soil in which they are raised, the amount of water they have received, and when they are gathered. Your recipes may not turn out exactly the same each time due to this differing potency.

For best results, follow these simple rules of drying and gathering herbs:

1. Gather herbs just before they flower (unless you are using the herb flower for your recipe, in which case gather the flowers when they are in full bloom). Gather plants and flowers during the day, while the sap is up.
2. Dry plants in an airy place in the shade. Hang them upside down to dry, then store them in jars when they are completely dry.
3. Gather roots in the fall, after the leaves are dead, or in the spring before the sap rises. Harvest roots in the evening, when the sap descends.
4. Gather bark in the fall or early spring.

COMMON NAME	SCIENTIFIC NAME	USE	COMMENTS
Alfalfa	*Medicago sativa*	Footbath, bath	Good source of vitamins C, D, E, K
Aloe	*Aloe vera*	Moisturizer, facial mask	Regenerates damaged tissue; good for burns and bruises
		Hair	Helps prevent dandruff

COMMON NAME	SCIENTIFIC NAME	USE	COMMENTS
Angelica	*Angelica archangelica*	Bath, herb pillow, potpourri	Oil of root used in bath
Anise seed	*Pimpinella anisum*	Toothpowder, body spritz, splasher	Freshens breath
Balm	*Melissa officinalis*	Facial steam, bath, herb pillows, potpourri	Cleanses skin
Basil	*Ocimum*	Hair preparations, bath, potpourri	Stimulating
Bay leaves	*Laurus nobilis*	Facial steam, bath, potpourri	Astringent, leaves soothes skin
Bergamot	*Monarda*	Hair preparations, bath, potpourri	Stimulates skin
Borage	*Borago officinalis*	Facial steam, facial mask	Good for dry, sensitive skin
Carnation	*Dianthus caryophyllus*	Potpourri	
Chamomile (Roman)	*Chamaemelum nobile*	Night cream	Strengthens and soothes skin
Chamomile (German)	*Matricaria rectutita*	Facial steam	Moisturizes, Penetrates skin
		Facial mask Eyewash, compress	Astringent, Antiseptic Anti-inflammatory; soothes

COMMON NAME	SCIENTIFIC NAME	USE	COMMENTS
Chamomile (German) *(cont'd)*		Hair preprations	Brightens fair hair; Softens all hair
		Bath	Moisturizes
		Insect lotion	
		Potpourri	
Cloves	*Syzygium aromaticum*	Footbath	Fights athlete foot fungi
		Toothpowder	Oil relieves toothache
		Potpourri	
Comfrey	*Symphytum officinale*	Night cream	Helps build tissues; restores cells
		Facial steam	Soothes and heals skin
		Toothpowder	Root used in toothpowder
		Bath	Keeps skin youthful
Elder flowers	*Sambucus nigra*	Splasher	Astringent
		Facial steam	Soothes, tightens skin
		Facial mask	Lightly bleaches skin
		Bath	
Eucalyptus	*Eucalyptus globulus*	Shampoo	Treats dandruff
		Moisturizer	Treats chapped skin; some individuals may be allergic
		Footbath, bath	Antiseptic
Eyebright flowers	*Euphrasia officinalis*	Splasher	Astringent, anti-inflammatory
		Eye compress	Soothes reddened eyes
Fennel seed	*Foeniculum vulgare*	Splasher	Cleans, refreshes skin

COMMON NAME	SCIENTIFIC NAME	USE	COMMENTS
Fennel Seed *(cont'd)*		Facial steam	Helps smooth lines away
		Facial mask	Softens the skin
		Eyewash	
Flax	*Linum usitatissimum*	Facial mask, hair preparations	Fibers make linen; seeds make linseed oil
Ginseng	*Panax*	Night cream	Helps delay aging process
Honey-suckle	*Lonicera periclymenum*	Potpourri	Fragrant, decorative
Hops	*Humulus lupulus*	Sleep pillow	Causes drowsiness
Horseradish	*Armoracia rusticana*	Facial mask	Heat-producing
Jasmine	*Jasminum*	Potpourri	Fragrant, decorative
Lady's mantle	*Alchemilla vulgaris*	Facial mask	Soothing skin tonic
Lavender	*Lavandula officinalis*	Splasher	Good for oily skin, acne
(English) (spike)	*L. angustifolia* *L. latifola*	Facial steam Bath, soap Potpourri, sachet	Stimulates the skin May cause allergic reactions in some individuals especially when exposed to sunlight; stimulating
Lemongrass	*Cymbopogon citratus*	Facial mask	
Lemon verbena	*Aloysia triphylla*	Bath, perfume, potpourri	Aromatic

COMMON NAME	SCIENTIFIC NAME	USE	COMMENTS
Licorice root	*Glycyrrhiza glabra*	Facial Steam	Soothes skin, opens pores
		Shampoo	Suppresses oil secretion in scalp
		Toothpowder, mouthwash	Freshens breath
Lily-of-the-valley	*Convallaria majalis*	Potpourri	Fragrant, decorative
Linden flowers	*Tilia americana*	Facial mask, bath	Softens the skin; soothing and relaxing
Lovage root	*Levisticum officinale*	Facial mask	Fades freckles
		Toothpaste	Sweetens breath
		Lotion	Cleanses and deodorizes
		Bath	Stimulating
Marigold	*Calendula officinalis*	Hair rinse	Brings out highlights
		Leg ointment	
		Foot powder	
		Bath	Antiseptic, astringent
Marjoram (wild)	*Origanum vulgare*	Hair rinse	Helps darken hair
		Bath	Antiseptic
(sweet)	*Origanum majorana*	Potpourri	
Mint	*Mentha*	Splasher	Astringent
(peppermint)	*Mentha piperita*	Facial steam, facial mask	Cools the skin; stimulates the skin
(spearmint)	*Mentha spicata*	Hair preparations	Conditions oily hair; controls dandruff
		Mouthwash	Freshens breath

COMMON NAME	SCIENTIFIC NAME	USE	COMMENTS
Mint (spearmint) *(cont'd)*		Bath	Restorative; too much in concentrated form can cause irritation
		Lotion	Clears chapped skin
		Potpourri	Fragrant
Mullein flowers	*Verbascum thapsus*	Hair preparations	Lightens the hair; intensifies blonde highlights
Orris	*Iris X germanica*	Herb pillow, potpourri	Fixative
Parsley	*Petroselinium crispum*	Splasher	Helps close large pores
		Facial steam	Freshens the skin
		Eye compress	Relieves puffiness
		Hair preparations	Makes dark hair shiny
		Mouthwash	Freshens breath
		Bath	
Rose petals, hips	*Rosa*	Facial steam	Softens and moisturizes
		Splasher	
		Eye Compress	
		Bath	perfumes the skin
		Lotion	
		Potpourri	
Rosemary	*Rosmarinus officinalis*	Facial steam, facial mask, hair preparations	Revitalizes, stimulates, and conditions scalp; prevents dandruff; encourages new growth
		Bath	Rejuvenating
			Helps circulation

COMMON NAME	SCIENTIFIC NAME	USE	COMMENTS
Rosemary *(cont'd)*		Potpourri, sachet	
Sage	*Salvia officinalis*	Splasher	Antiseptic
(Clary)	*Salvia scalera*	Moisturizer, neck cream	Cleanses the skin
		Facial steam	Astringent, refresher
		Facial mask	Closes large pores
		Hair preparations	Prevents hair from graying; refreshes the hair
		Mouthwash	Deodorizes
Salad Burnet	*Poterium sanguisorba*	Bath	
Savory (summer)	*Satureja hortensis*	Mouthwash	Freshens breath
Shavegrass (horsetail)	*Equisetum*	Facial mask	Skin tonic
Southern-wood	*Artemisia abrotanum*	Hair preparations Potpourri	Restorative
Stinging nettle	*Urtica dioica*	Hair preparations	Handle with gloves until boiling water has been poured over the herb; infusions are used to stimulate growth of hair and to treat dandruff
		Facial mask	Astringent
		Bath	Increases circulation

COMMON NAME	SCIENTIFIC NAME	USE	COMMENTS
Thyme	*Thymus vulgaris*	Facial steam	Good for normal skin; helps tone up the skin; has antiseptic and disinfectant qualities
		Hair preparations Mouthwash Footbath, bath Lotion	Freshens breath Soothes the skin, calms the nerves
Watercress	*Nasturtium officinale*	Splasher Mouthwash	Good for blemishes Freshens breath
Yarrow leaves	*Achillea millefolium*	Facial steam Facial mask Lotions	Astringent Cleansing

Appendix C: Glossary

alcohol   An antiseptic astringent used in cosmetics. Very drying.

astringent   A substance such as alcohol used to tighten the skin. Generally used on oily skin.

baking soda   A water soluble substance available in supermarkets used in baths as a soothing soak for itchy, irritated skin. Also used as a simple toothpaste.

beeswax   A substance secreted by bees that is used in cosmetics to soften and protect the skin.

castile soap   Soap made from at least 40 percent olive oil.

castor oil   Oil from the castor bean. An emollient that forms a hard film when dry, it is often used in cosmetics such as lipsticks.

cereals   Starchy grain products such as bran, cornmeal, wheat germ, and oatmeal. These should be used in raw form.

cocoa butter   A solid fat from the cacao bean used to soften and lubricate the skin and to harden creams.

coconut oil   Fat obtained from coconut that melts at body temperature used to soften and lubricate the skin.

cornstarch   A slick, slightly abrasive starch obtained from corn kernels that is used as a powder for irritated skin.

decoction   Liquid made by placing herbs in cold water and bringing to a boil, then simmering, cooling, and straining.

essential oil   The "essence" of the plant, concentrated aromatic oils obtained through various processes. They are sometimes mixed with carrier oils or can be diluted in alcohol solutions. Use sparingly, because they are very potent.

extracts   Concentrated form of substances.

gel   A jellylike material such as the clear innards of an aloe leaf.

gelatin Animal protein extracted from hooves, bones, and tendons used in cosmetics because it adheres to skin and hair.

honey A sweet, sticky substance made by honeybees from flower nectar used for external skin problems and in cosmetics as an astringent and moisturizer. Each flower produces honey that is unique in flavor and color.

infusion Liquid made by pouring boiling water over herbs or by adding herbs to boiling water, removing from heat and letting steep, then straining.

insoluble Not able to be dissolved.

lanolin Oil obtained from wool that is used in cosmetics to prevent or relieve excess skin dryness.

moisturizer Any substance that adds moisture to the skin.

pH A scale ranging from 0 to 14 that measures the acidity or alkalinity of a substance. Vinegar, (pH 2.3), honey, skin, and hair are acid. Most soaps (pH 8 to 10) and mineral waters are alkaline. Plain water is either neutral (pH 7) or very close to neutral.

poultice A soft, usually heated and sometimes medicated, moist compress applied to sore or inflamed parts of the body.

rose water A watery solution made of the odiferous parts of the rose used as perfume. It can be obtained by simmering roses and water together and collecting the steam distillate or by infusing pure oil of roses in distilled water for a number of days and then discarding the oil by straining.

soluble May be dissolved.

steep Soak in a liquid.

tepid Temperature of a liquid that is moderately warm.

Appendix D: Sources

If you cannot find ingredients locally, here are some mail-order sources.

Earth Reverence
5615 41st Avenue East
Bradenton, FL 34208
813/748-1659
Catalog is $2.50, refundable on first order (minimum $25).

Haussmann's Pharmacy
534–536 West Girard Avenue
Philadelphia, PA 19123
215/627-2143 or
800/235-5522

Herb & Spice
PO Box 299
Norway, IA 52318
319/227-7996 or
800/786-1388

Herb 'n' Renewal
Rural Route 1
Laura, IL 61451
309/639-4145

Long Creek Herbs
Route 4, Box 730
Oak Grove, AR 72660
417/779-5450
Catalog is $2, refundable on first order.

Mountain Rose Herbs
PO Box 2000
Redway, CA 95560
707/923-3941 or
800/879-3337
Catalog is $1.

Swanson Health Products
Box 2803
Fargo, ND 58108-2803
800/437-4148

Tom's of Maine
106 LaFayette Center
Kennebunk, ME 04043
207/985-3874

$\mathcal{I}_{NDEX}$